AF781123

Comprehensive Guide to Müller-'

John Wong-Chung

# Comprehensive Guide to Müller-Weiss Disease

Springer

John Wong-Chung
Ulster Independent Clinic
Belfast, Northern Ireland, UK

School of Medicine
Ulster University
Londonderry, Northern Ireland, UK

ISBN 978-3-031-66643-8 ISBN 978-3-031-66644-5 (eBook)
https://doi.org/10.1007/978-3-031-66644-5

© The Editor(s) (if applicable) and The Author(s), under exclusive license to Springer Nature Switzerland AG 2024

This work is subject to copyright. All rights are solely and exclusively licensed by the Publisher, whether the whole or part of the material is concerned, specifically the rights of translation, reprinting, reuse of illustrations, recitation, broadcasting, reproduction on microfilms or in any other physical way, and transmission or information storage and retrieval, electronic adaptation, computer software, or by similar or dissimilar methodology now known or hereafter developed.
The use of general descriptive names, registered names, trademarks, service marks, etc. in this publication does not imply, even in the absence of a specific statement, that such names are exempt from the relevant protective laws and regulations and therefore free for general use.
The publisher, the authors and the editors are safe to assume that the advice and information in this book are believed to be true and accurate at the date of publication. Neither the publisher nor the authors or the editors give a warranty, expressed or implied, with respect to the material contained herein or for any errors or omissions that may have been made. The publisher remains neutral with regard to jurisdictional claims in published maps and institutional affiliations.

This Springer imprint is published by the registered company Springer Nature Switzerland AG
The registered company address is: Gewerbestrasse 11, 6330 Cham, Switzerland

If disposing of this product, please recycle the paper.

*I dedicate this, my first textbook, to my first wife who has tolerated the numerous countless hours spent not only at the hospital, but researching and writing on the computer, a.k.a. the second wife.*

# Foreword

It gives me great pleasure to introduce *Comprehensive Guide to Müller-Weiss Disease*. It is the first truly comprehensive textbook on this condition. This condition is complex, to say the least. There are only a few papers published based on a large cohort of patients in the International literature on this subject. These usually involve classifications which do not necessarily help the individual surgeon as to how to treat and manage this condition. So it comes as a "breath of fresh air" that somebody has written a comprehensive text on this subject based on his large series. The author I have known since we were colleagues in medical school. Since then, he and I trained and become Consultant Orthopaedic Foot and Ankle Surgeons. Over the years, I have noted his diligence and enquiring nature into orthopaedic Foot and Ankle problems.

This book brings together all what is known about Müller-Weiss Disease published in the International literature and then developed by his own large experience of treating patients with this condition. It certainly clarifies the condition, as much as it can, with our present knowledge. It does however, with his own classification which is published, guide the reader into an appropriate treatment programme. However, being the condition that it is, it then stimulates the reader to consider what further research can be done to move forward our knowledge on this condition. The number of patients with this condition is relatively small worldwide. There is nothing that is better than a book that tells the history of a disease and the hypotheses that relate to its aetiology. Treatment programmes will assist the reader of this book to manage the condition. However, more importantly, it may stimulate the way forward to develop a greater understanding which I am sure will require significant global collaboration between large Foot and Ankle Orthopaedic surgical centres.

Dublin, Ireland<br>February 2024

Professor Michael M. Stephens, M.Sc. (BioEng.), FRCSI<br>Founding Editor, *Foot and Ankle Surgery*

# Preface

Writing a book demands as much effort and perseverance, if not more than writing a research paper for publication. Why write? An internet search reveals the many purposes of writing: (1) to inform, (2) to express, (3) to describe, (4) to explore and learn, (5) to explain, (6) to argue, (7) to persuade, (8) to evaluate, (9) to problem solve, (10) to mediate and (11) to entertain.

So, why a book on Müller-Weiss disease? While not initially recognizing what the condition was in the first case that presented to our service, we subsequently published on 19 feet—marking the beginning of our journey to *inform* with "Recognition and Management of Müller-Weiss Disease" in *Foot and Ankle International* in 2012. Nine years later, the number of feet diagnosed at our unit with Müller-Weiss disease rose to 68. In "Radiographic Analysis of Müller-Weiss Disease" published in *Foot and Ankle Surgery* in 2021, we *explored, learnt and argued* that the heel was not always in varus as previously purported by Spanish investigators. And by 2023, an extensive province-wide analysis of radiographs of 95 feet enabled formulation of a grouping system. Published in July 2023 in *Foot and Ankle Surgery*, "Towards Understanding Müller-Weiss Disease from an Analysis of 95 Cases" aimed to *problem solve* through provision of a standardized platform for reporting and studying the condition and its treatment. The last article in press in the Journal of *Foot and Ankle Surgery* at the time of writing, "Outcomes of Selective Arthrodesis Based on Joints Affected in 33 Feet with Müller-Weiss Disease," reports the author's experience with selective arthrodesis surgery based on the joints involved. It was actually meant to be the second, but only achieved peer review acceptance this year.

The purpose of this book then is to continue with the same mission—to *inform, describe, explore and learn, explain, evaluate, argue* and *problem solve*—towards defining gold standards in the treatment of Müller-Weiss disease. Perforce, a book grants the author a certain degree of *carte blanche,* to *express* personal views, even *persuade* a little and in choosing what to write—including perhaps some thought processes deemed provocative by some but intended to stimulate further research, discussion and brainstorming.

This book shares the author's journey with a relatively rare condition, which somehow is frequent in Northern Ireland, particularly in the North-West.

In addition, it includes a comprehensive and critical review of the recent barrage of literature available on the subject. Each reference has been carefully scrutinized and its essence distilled into this book. The chapters are purposefully short and concise for easy reading. Illustrations are provided to complement the written description. Where relevant, diagrams are included to give the readership a wide picture of what authors worldwide are describing, with the aim of reaching a universal common platform, for there also appears to be geographical differences in distribution and pathology.

The last chapter entitled "Past, Present and Future Directions" summarizes controversies surrounding aetiology, classification, obligatory heel varus and the array of different procedures advocated in its surgical management. It emphasizes the need for a common platform when reporting disease outcomes. It ends with a list of numerous questions and unknowns that remain to be answered and suggestions for future areas of research.

The overarching aims of this book are to advance understanding of a disease which we still do not fully comprehend, from its aetiology to its classification, and in so doing create pathways to determine its optimum management.

We are all born. We go to Primary School, Secondary School, College, University and then to the Workplace. As we advance through these stages, we are often unaware of the people who truly made a difference in our lives. Until we have passed through these life's stages, that is.

I take this opportunity to gratefully acknowledge the important people who shaped my Education, without which this book would never have reached fruition. Starting from Primary School, Monsieur Charlotte and Miss Nadeige Rosette taught me French and English Grammar and Comprehension. In Secondary School, Monsieur Georges Espitalier-Noël taught me English Literature and essay writing, besides being a great source of life inspiration. Monsieur Wan Hok Chee (Maths), Monsieur Roger Perdreau (Chemistry) and Monsieur Sultan (Physics) transferred their unique styles of teaching and learning, which have served me throughout the rest of university and working life. Professor Tim O'Brien and Dr. Munro Strong encouraged and coached me in Research and writing in Scientific English. I also thank my mentors, Martin Walsh and Frank McManus for their help and support during and after my training years.

I also acknowledge the support of Alistair Wilson, who has provided selfless guidance throughout my journey in *Foot and Ankle Surgery*; the Orthopaedic Residents, Raymond McKenna, Andrew Walls, Matthew Lynch-Wong, Andrew Blythe and Matthew Arneill; Liam Fleming, Physical Therapist; and Elaine Lynch, Physician Associate—all of whom patiently listened to my ramblings about Müller-Weiss disease throughout the past few years. And finally, Michael Stephens, the grandfather of the Irish Orthopaedic Foot and Ankle Society (IOFAS), who has supported my works and efforts throughout the years.

My sincere hope is that this book will be of service to the Health Professionals who treat Foot and Ankle conditions and in turn benefit those who suffer from Müller-Weiss disease.

Belfast/Londonderry, UK Professor John Wong-Chung

# Contents

# List of Figures

# List of Tables

# Abbreviations

| | |
|---|---|
| 3-D | Three-dimensional |
| 4-corners | Junction between anterior calcaneal process, inferolateral border of talar head, lateral edge of navicular and superior border of cuboid. |
| AO | Arbeitsgemeinschaft für osteosynthesefragen |
| AOFAS | American Orthopaedic Foot and Ankle Society |
| AP | Anteroposterior |
| ATP | Association of Tennis Professionals |
| BMAC | Bone marrow aspirate concentrate |
| BMI | Body mass index |
| BOFAS | British Orthopaedic Foot and Ankle Society |
| CC | Calcaneocuboid |
| CT | Computerized axial tomography |
| CTEV | Congenital talipes equinovarus |
| Double medial | Arthrodesis of subtalar and talonavicular joints |
| DPTFM | Dorsoplantar talo-first metatarsal angle |
| FAOS | Foot and Ankle Outcome Score |
| IOFAS | Irish Orthopaedic Foot and Ankle Society |
| IQR | Interquartile range |
| JSSF | Japanese Society for Surgery of the Foot |
| LDCO | Lateral displacement calcaneal osteotomy |
| MRI | Magnetic resonance imaging |
| MTP | Metatarsophalangeal |
| MWD | Müller-Weiss disease |
| NC | Naviculocuneiform |
| NC1 | Medial naviculocuneiform joint |
| NC2 | Middle naviculocuneiform joint |
| NC3 | Lateral naviculocuneiform joint |
| NORD | National Organization for Rare Diseases |
| NSAID | Non-steroidal anti-inflammatory drugs |
| OLT | Osteochondral lesion of talus |
| PCFD | Progressive collapsing foot deformity |

| | |
|---|---|
| POA | Preoperative assessment clinic |
| SamJap | Save as many Joints as Possible |
| SPECT-CT | Singe-photon emission computed tomography |
| STIR | Short tau inversion recovery |
| Tc | Technetium |
| TICBG | Tricortical iliac crest bone graft |
| TMT | Tarsometatarsal |
| TN | Talonavicular |
| TNC | Talonaviculocuneiform |
| VAS | Visual Analog Scale |
| WBCT | Weight-bearing CT scan |
| WHO | World Health Organization |
| Wong | Wong-Chung |

G capitalized in Group when followed by a number, e.g. Group 1, Group 2 and Group 3.
S capitalized in Stage when followed by a Roman numeral, e.g. Stage I, Stage II, etc.

# Part I
# Analysis of Elemental Facts in Müller-Weiss Disease

# Chapter 1
# Aetiology to Nomenclature

**Abstract** Müller-Weiss disease is an affliction primarily of the navicular bone with secondary involvement of the perinavicular joints. Its exact aetiology remains undetermined despite proposal of various theories. Current consensus is that an overlong second metatarsal or first ray brachymetatarsia leads to eccentric compression of the lateral portion of the navicular. A comma-shaped navicular results with medial extrusion of its medial pole, medial talonavicular subluxation and lateral shift of the talar head. Delayed ossification arising from nutritional deficiency was once considered another major factor predisposing a weakened navicular to deformation under eccentric loading. Another element, as yet unidentified, must be responsible since not all index minus feet go on to develop Müller-Weiss disease. It is not a bipartite navicular as true partitioning produces two fragments of equal size that do not wander from their normal location. Severe forms of Brailsford's osteochondritis and 'bipartite navicular' represent advanced stages of the disease, whereby fragmentation of the lateral navicular occurs, marked medial extrusion of its medial pole and dorsal displacement of the lateral navicular fragment ensue, leaving room for the talar head to articulate directly with the lateral cuneiform bone forming the so-called talocuneiform articulation that characterizes Maceira end-stage V disease.

**Keywords** Müller-Weiss disease · Navicular · Delayed ossification · Index-minus metatarsal formula · Brailsford's osteochondritis · Bipartite navicular

## Introduction

Despite the numerous theories proposed since its first description almost a century ago, the precise aetiology of Müller-Weiss disease still remains unclear. To compound matters, there has been considerable variation in the way it has been reported over the years throughout different parts of the world.

This Chapter seeks to elucidate the timeline of the various theories and terminologies applied to this relatively rare condition.

© The Author(s), under exclusive license to Springer Nature Switzerland AG 2024

J. Wong-Chung, *Comprehensive Guide to Müller-Weiss Disease*,
https://doi.org/10.1007/978-3-031-66644-5_1

## 1.1 Definition

Müller-Weiss disease is an affliction primarily of the navicular bone with secondary involvement of the perinavicular joints.

## 1.2 Anatomical Considerations

### 1.2.1 *Vascular Supply of the Navicular*

- Medial plantar artery supplies the plantar and part of the medial aspect of the navicular.
- Dorsalis pedis artery supplies the dorsal and lateral one third of the navicular.
- Navicular tuberosity is supplied by an anastomosis between medial plantar and dorsalis pedis arteries.
- The central zone, which is also the area of maximum shear stress, has a relatively poor blood supply as demonstrated by microangiography in fresh cadavers (Torg et al. 1982). Its vascularity may decrease even further with age.

### 1.2.2 *Anatomy*

The talar head articulates with the "acetabulum pedis", the bony boundaries of which are the posterior articular facet of the navicular anteriorly, and the anterior and middle facets of the subtalar joint inferiorly. The soft tissue envelope includes the superomedial portion of the spring ligament medially and the inferolateral portion of the spring ligament in the floor, supplemented laterally by the calcaneonavicular component of the bifurcate ligament.

### 1.2.3 *Biomechanics*

The navicular is the keystone of the medial column of the foot. It contributes to the integrity of both medial longitudinal and transverse arches of the foot. The 'acetabulum pedis' or talocalcaneonavicular articulation is responsible for almost 80% of motion at the hindfoot. Together with the naviculocuneiform joints, it bears the greatest load transmission compared to other foot joints, during the second and third rockers of gait.

## 1.3 Eponyms

The condition is named after Walther Müller and Konrad Weiss who both independently described the condition in 1927. Müller, surgeon in Leipzig, initially believed compressive forces had caused a mechanical collapse in an 18-year-old girl, but a year later proposed a congenital cause instead (Müller 1927). Weiss, an Austrian radiologist, working with Robert Kienböck renowned for describing avascular necrosis of the lunate, believed it was an osteonecrotic process (Weiss 1927).

Despite the eponyms, Georg Schmidt reportedly described the first case in 1925 in association with pluriglandular insufficiency, but did not provide images of his patient.

Müller-Weiss disease is sometimes referred to as Brailsford disease, after James F. Brailsford (1888–1961) (Brailsford 1935a, b, 1939, 1953). He was a Sergeant Radiographer in the British Army during World War I. After the war ended, he joined Birmingham Medical School at the age of 30 years. He founded the British Association of Radiologists, of which he was the first President. He authored the classic textbook "The Radiology of Bones and Joints" in 1934. He is also well known for his 1929 description of a rare form of skeletal dysplasia, Morquio-Brailsford syndrome.

## 1.4 Terminology

Its exact aetiology remains undetermined. Numerous theories have been proposed. As a result, different terminologies have been applied to this condition creating considerable confusion that persists to date. Named after Müller and Weiss, some call it Brailsford's disease, after Brailsford who believed it represented an osteochondritis (Brailsford 1935a, b, 1939, 1953; Sharp et al. 2003). Others refer to it as a bipartite navicular (Volk 1937; Zimmer 1938; Fine 1941; Hatoff 1950; Mau 1960; Wiley and Brown 1981; Shawdon et al. 1995; Tanaka et al. 2006; Yamaguchi et al. 2016; Chujo et al. 2023).

Wiley and Brown, Tanaka et al. accept interchangeable use of the terms, implying synonymity of the four appellations—Müller-Weiss disease, Brailsford's disease, osteochondritis and bipartite navicular (Wiley and Brown 1981; Tanaka et al. 2006). On the other hand, Yamaguchi et al. believe bipartite navicular and osteochondritis represent the same condition affecting a younger age group while Müller-Weiss disease is a different entity occurring in middle-aged adults with advanced arthritis (Yamaguchi et al. 2016).

## 1.5 Aetiology

Consensus hence needs to be reached as to whether these four designations refer to the same condition. In the meantime, the numerous theories proposed in the aetiology of conditions variously known as Müller-Weiss disease, Brailsford's disease, osteochondritis and bipartite navicular, will now be expounded upon, irrespective of actual cause which remains unknown.

In view of the frequent citations in the literature, Brailsford's disease, osteochondritis and bipartite navicular will be elaborated upon in greater detail before final discussion of contemporary theories behind what is now known as Müller-Weiss disease.

### *1.5.1 Normal Variant*

In the discussion of bipartite navicular, Shawdon et al. (Australia, 1995) had considered whether it represented a normal variant (Shawdon et al. 1995).

### *1.5.2 Trauma*

In 1935, Brailsford had attributed formation of a bipartite navicular to either a single or repeated episodes of trauma (Brailsford 1935a). Wiley and Brown alluded to a 22-year-old man who sustained a fracture of the navicular in a head-on car collision (Wiley and Brown 1981). Pattern of fracture displacement was the same as with a bipartite navicular, the lateral fragment displacing dorsolaterally while the medial fragment displaced medially and inferiorly. However, they thought it unlikely that a traumatic incident could produce such similar and consistent deformities as with a bipartite navicular. Trauma would also not account for bilaterality as in some cases. Furthermore, none of their 6 cases gave a history of trauma.

### *1.5.3 Abnormal Evolution of Köhler's Disease*

Brailsford recounted on a 12-year-old boy, whose initial diagnosis of Köhler's disease was published in the first edition of his textbook, and who developed osteochondritis 6 years later (Brailsford 1939). However, Wiley and Brown found no evidence to suggest Köhler's disease could leave residual deformity (Wiley and Brown 1981).

### 1.5.4 *Brailsford's Disease—Osteochondritis*

The works by Brailsford deserve highlighting and in-depth description (Brailsford 1935a, b, 1953, 1939).

In 1939, Brailsford published on 18 feet in 9 bilateral cases of osteochondritis affecting the navicular in adult women only with 'compression and division of the bone and subsequent listhesis of the separated fragments' (Brailsford 1939). He had previously reported on 5 cases in 1935, when he had cited trauma as cause of disease (Brailsford 1935a). His introduction opens with a description of Köhler's disease as an affection of children between the age of 2½ and 10 years old. It affects predominantly boys aged 5–6 years old and ends with complete clinical and radiological recovery, 1½ to 4 years later.

The youngest patient, a 22-year-old nurse, complained of pain and swelling over the mid-dorsal aspect of both feet, worse towards the end of a working day. Radiographs of the left foot revealed compression of the lateral half of the navicular to about two-thirds of the thickness of the normal medial half. Superiorly lay a 'small sequestrated fragment' akin to a 'loose body in the medial femoral condyle in osteochondritis dissecans', which led Brailsford to refer to the disease as an osteochondritis. Radiological changes were more marked at the right foot where the navicular 'had been severed obliquely into two parts through its middle third.' The lateral fragment was displaced dorsally and distally to override the lateral cuneiform, its distal surface lying level with the base of the fourth metatarsal. 'The medial half appeared to be squeezed between the head of the astragalus and the first and second cuneiforms.' It had 'glided in a proximal direction over the medial surface of the head of the astragalus'. The thickness of the navicular had halved at the level of the middle cuneiform. On lateral roentgenogram, a cleft ran from the dorsal distal surface of the navicular to the midpoint of the talonavicular joint. The medial fragment tended to override the dorsal surface of the adjacent medial cuneiform, which looked moulded by pressure. Serial radiographs over a 5-year period demonstrated slight gradual increase in compression of the lateral half of the left navicular and gradually increasing right medial talonavicular subluxation, but with no secondary arthritic changes. She was prescribed exercises and continued to work as a nurse.

The second patient, a 32-year-old woman with no history of injury, was initially diagnosed with tibialis anterior tendinitis. Radiographs showed similar bilateral changes with oblique division of the navicular into 2 parts through its middle third, a greater degree of medial talonavicular subluxation and a resulting greater degree of separation of the fragments, overriding of the lateral fragment over the dorsum of the lateral cuneiform and early signs of arthritis at the right foot. 'The second metatarsal of each foot showed hypertrophy while the fourth and fifth metatarsals were slender.'

The third woman, aged 52 years old, displayed the characteristic splitting of the left navicular. The medial fragment had 'slipped so far medially that more than half of its articular surface projected beyond the articular surface of the head of the astragalus'. The longitudinal axis of the first metatarsal passed medial to the inner surface of the talar neck instead of through its mid-axis. In effect, Brailsford was describing over 50% of medial talonavicular subluxation and an alteration of the dorsoplantar talo-first metarsal angle indicative of midfoot abduction. The first metatarsals were short. The second metatarsals were hypertrophied, while the third, fourth and fifth were atrophied. Six years later, severe osteoarthritis had developed at the left talonavicular joint. The lateral fragment had displaced completely over the dorsum of the adjacent cuneiform. At the contralateral right foot, the lateral third of the navicular was compressed with no splitting, as with the left foot of the first patient.

The fourth case, a 45-year-old woman had bilateral splitting of the navicular with even more marked medial talonavicular subluxation and midfoot abduction, such that the axes of both first and second metatarsals passed well medial to the inner surface of the talus. Severe talonavicular osteoarthritis was present, more marked on the right side, where the calcaneocuboid joint was also arthritic. The first metatarsals were short with hypertrophy of the second and atrophy of the third, fourth and fifth metatarsals.

The fifth case, a 52-year-old woman with bilateral splitting of the navicular, had the most severe degree of talonavicular subluxation and advanced arthritis including at the left calcaneocuboid joint. There was neither shortness of the first metatarsal nor hypertrophy of the second, but the third, fourth and fifth metatarsals were atrophied.

The sixth case, a 56-year-old woman, had the least displacement and deformity with near normal looking metatarsals except for osteoporosis of the fifth. Secondary degenerative changes were seen at the deformed joints.

The seventh, a 57-year-old woman had always had severe valgus deformity of the left foot. The medial arch sagged. There was complete medial displacement of the navicular over the talar head with some accompanying forefoot adduction and severe talonavicular arthritis. Arthritic changes were also present at the first tarsometatarsal and calcaneocuboid joints. Slight changes were seen at the right foot, similar to the contralateral foot in the first and third patients.

The eighth, a 59-year-old woman gave a doubtful history of injury 9 years previously. Radiographs showed the characteristic deformity of the navicular in both feet with marked medial talonavicular subluxation and arthritis on the right side.

The ninth, a 51-year-old woman had the characteristic deformity of the navicular with marked medial talonavicular subluxation and collapse of the medial arch. Changes were less severe on the left side.

Brailsford found no men with comparable roentgenographic appearances. However, in several men, all of whom gave a history of injury, changes in the navicular appeared similar to Kienböck's disease of the lunate. A 33-year-old male laborer was claiming compensation for a foot injury sustained from a fall off a ladder 2 months previously. Clinical diagnosis was of a fractured metatarsal. On lateral radiography, the navicular displayed changes akin to a Kienböck's lunatomalacia. Dorsoplantar radiograph suggested separation into 2 parts through the middle third of the navicular. Overall appearances were so like those of another patient with no history of injury, entered 2 years prior in the author's collection of cases with Kienböck's lunatomalacia, that they could have been mistaken for the same patient. As there was no sign of disease in the contralateral navicular, and from a study of serial radiographs following navicular fractures in other patients, Brailsford was 'satisfied' the findings in the 33-year-old man represented post fracture changes. In another 51-year-old man, with no history of injury, unusual deformity of the navicular and changes in the talar head noted in each foot were suggestive of osteochondritis.

In 9 patients, all women, aged 22–59 (mean, 47.3) years old, Brailsford summarized his findings thus. Oblique splitting of the navicular occurred with separation of the 2 fragments. The medial fragment gradually glided over the head of the astragalus towards its medial side, while the lateral fragment overrode the dorsal surface of the middle and lateral cuneiforms. The resultant gap between the 2 navicular fragments effectively reduced the distance between the talar head and proximal surfaces of the middle and lateral cuneiform bones. Eventually, the talar head articulated directly with the middle and lateral cuneiforms in some cases. Severe osteoarthritis ensued at the mid-tarsal joints in later stages of the disease.

Disease was bilateral, with less extensive changes on one side such as osteochondritis or 'mere compression of the plastic outer third of the navicular'. In the 2 younger patients, there was no secondary arthritis whereas in all the other older feet, marked osteoarthritic changes became evident. In the third woman aged 52 years old, there was almost complete medial talonavicular dislocation with no detectable secondary degeneration. Six years later, severe arthritic changes had ensued, suggesting that displacement had probably occurred within a year or so of the first radiographic examination.

In 3 patients, Cases 2, 3 and 4, the first metatarsal was short. The second was hypertrophied. The third, fourth and fifth were atrophied. These features were not seen in the others, although some atrophy of the metatarsals was present in Cases 5 and 7.

Unfortunately, the quality of reproduction of the radiographs dating back so many years ago, does not permit critical evaluation. Nevertheless, the written description of the radiological findings is remarkably accurate and precise. They match and antedate that of Maceira and Rochera by 65 years (Maceira and Rochera 2004). Brailsford's radiographic description from the early part of the last century is truly outstanding in that little else can be added to it, 84 years on. By 1945, Brailsford's collection increased to 17 cases and by 1953, he had collected 20 cases altogether for the fifth edition of his textbook (Brailsford 1953).

### *1.5.5 Bipartite Navicular*

The topic of bipartite navicular also deserves further elaboration. Its timeline (1937) closely parallels that of Brailsford's disease (1935). And so do their descriptions. It also only became recognized after introduction of roentgenography. In 1937, Volk reported on 2 cases of bipartite navicular (Volk 1937). The following year, Zimmer published on a 19-year-old patient (Zimmer 1938). On the dorsoplantar view, the smaller fragment appeared comma-shaped and lay superimposed on the medial two cuneiforms and the main navicular fragment. On the lateral view, the smaller fragment was triangular and situated dorsally. It was separated from the main fragment by a cleft directed upwards and anteriorly. No disease could be identified histologically (Coughlin 2007; Sarrafian 2011).

In 1941, de Fine Licht reported on 2 bilateral cases (Fine 1941). On dorsoplantar roentgenogram, the smaller fragment appeared wedge-shaped, with its base medial and its apex directed laterally. On the lateral view, the same fragment looked wedge-shaped with its apex plantar. Sporadic case reports emerged in 1950 and 1960 (Hatoff 1950; Mau 1960). Shawdon and Kiss (1995) described its CT appearances, wedge-shaped with tapering margins, as distinct from an acute or stress fracture (Shawdon et al. 1995).

Wiley and Brown (Ontario, Canada, 1981) acknowledged Brailsford's description of an uncommon entity characterized by 'bipartition' of the navicular, displacement and separation of the two fragments, 'listhesis of the tarsal scaphoid' and its association with flatfoot (Wiley and Brown 1981). They published another 6 patients, 3 of whom had bilateral involvement, aged 8 to 53 (mean, 24.67 ± 18.89) years old. There were 4 male and 2 female patients. Four were aged below 16 years old, which is not surprising considering that Wiley was based at Children's Hospital of Eastern Ontario. None gave a history of trauma. All feet were painful except for the opposite foot in a 16-year-old boy. The latter was thought to have peroneal muscle spasm on the painful side. All presented with painful flatfoot, except for a 44-year-old woman, who complained of pain but had no flatfoot. All exhibited some degree of stiffness of the subtalar and midtarsal joints.

Radiographic findings were consistent in each case. On dorsoplantar views, the dorsal fragment had displaced laterally and appeared superimposed over the middle and lateral cuneiforms. The medial fragment had subluxated medially and plantarwards, around the talar head. In that position, it was thought to have moved closer to the medial cuneiform. On lateral radiographs, an oblique cleft ran from dorsal distal to plantar proximal, separating the smaller dorsolateral fragment from the remainder of the navicular bone. Wiley thought that this divergent displacement of the two navicular fragments was what Brailsford was referring to as 'listhesis'. The latter term is derived from the Greek word, *olistháno͂* which means 'to slip, to slide, to glide'. There was no radiological evidence of avascular necrosis. Nor was there evidence of adjacent bone or joint involvement other than expected degenerative changes at the site of lesion. No further displacement occurred at follow-up.

The 44-year-old woman, who had a long-standing varus deformity of the hindfoot, underwent triple arthrodesis with a satisfactory result. Otherwise, they did not advocate any specific treatment other than symptomatic management. According to Wiley and Brown, Brailsford and Müller were describing the same entity as a bipartite navicular.

Wiley and Brown acknowledged that 4 of their patients were under the age of 16 years. They postulated that the lesion existed in childhood and remained unrecognised until there were significant signs and symptoms. Deformity only became apparent after the bipartite fragments separated, producing a rather large medial prominence that simulated a pes planus deformity. Eventually, degenerative changes set in with pain and stiffness. These changes were thought to begin early in life.

### Navicular Partitioning in Horses

Interestingly, bipartite and even tripartite navicular has been described in horses. Van der Zaag et al. (2016) reported on a bipartite navicular in the left forelimb of a 10-year-old Belgian Warmblood gelding, a tripartite navicular in both forelimbs of a 7-year-old Quarter Horse stallion with chronic degenerative and cystic changes, and a bipartite navicular in the left hindlimb of a 5-year-old Dutch Warmblood gelding (Zaag et al. 2016). There was no mention of relative metatarsal lengths or radiographs showing the metatarsals in relation to the navicular.

The authors were aware of the more frequent reports of bipartite navicular and its theories in human medical literature. Considered as an anatomical variant by some, others believed it resulted from failure of fusion of ossification centres or from formation of an extra aberrant ossification centre.

In horses, the location of partitioning is consistently uniform at one-third of the length of the bone, either at its medial or lateral wing, in the 'para-sagittal' plane. In case of tripartition, the 2 partitions are evenly spread along the entire length of the same bone, which makes it unlikely to represent evenly distributed parallel fractures.

Rijkenhuizen et al. (1989) had shown that certain parts of the equine navicular receive arteries from only one side while other parts received blood supply from more than one direction. Van der Zaag (2016) thought that parts supplied by one artery were more susceptible to ischemia, thereby predisposing these zones to partitioning during foetal development rather than during adult life, with ensuing disorders of enchondral ossification. The sites of partition seemed to correspond with the junctions of regions receiving one artery and regions with multiple blood supply. The authors concluded that bipartition or tripartition represented a congenital condition caused by vascular disturbance during foetal growth. In the adult horse, chronic repetitive biomechanical stress may then induce local degeneration with subchondral cyst formation leading to lameness.

Macroscopically, the continuous smooth lining of articular cartilage deviates into the bone at the site of partition. There is no complete separation or displacement of the fragments, unlike as in the human so-called bipartite navicular.

### The Case Against Partitioning of the Navicular in Humans

Phylogenetically, two tarsal ossification centers, comparable in site to the navicular, can be found in certain primitive reptiles. In mammals, the tibiale of the first ray forms the accessory navicular or os tibiale externum (Fig. 1.1). The distal tibial and fibular centrale of the second and third rays form the body of the navicular (Sarrafian 2011).

According to Trolle (1948), a true bipartition would produce 2 bones with similar sizes, which together would equal the size of a normal navicular. Also, the 2 fragments would both be in relatively normal anatomical location. In the human so-called bipartite navicular and in Müller-Weiss disease, the 2 fragments are unequal in size. The loose navicular fragment does not remain in normal anatomical position. It

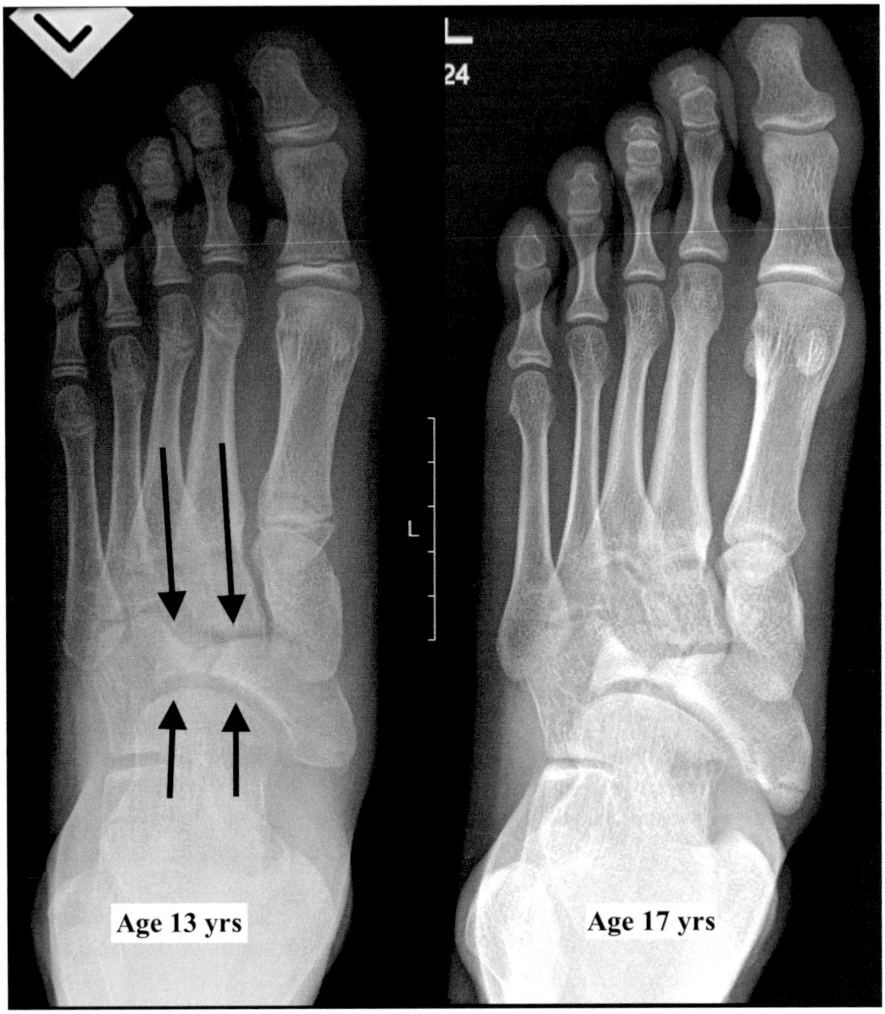


**Fig. 1.1** Dorsoplantar radiographs of a boy with early-onset Group 1 Müller-Weiss disease at age 13 and 17 years old. Note cortical hypertrophy of the second metatarsal, which is longer than the first. The third metatarsal appears relatively hypertrophied also. Hypotrophy of the fourth more than the first and fifth metatarsals. Compression and fragmentation of the lateral navicular with medial extrusion of the medial navicular pole. The talar head has shifted laterally with decrease in Kite's angle. All metatarsals lie remarkably parallel to each other. The sesamoids sit in 'too pretty' position beneath the first metatarsal head. Arrows indicate increased stress forces acting upon the lateral navicular between the talar head and middle/lateral cuneiform bone duo from overlong second ray. The tiny accessory navicular bone at age 13 years has grown in size by age 17 years. The 3 pieces of bone are all unequal in size and not uniformly distributed

displaces dorsally and laterally. In horses, partitioning in horses is symmetrical and does not result in separation of the fragments. Wiley and Brown (1981) had considered another possibility, that of heterogenous ossification centres rather than true bipartition.

### *1.5.6 Migration of Accessory Cuboid*

In the discussion of bipartite navicular, de Fine Licht thought it conceivable that the lateral fragment that is found displaced dorsally and laterally to overlie the lateral cuneiform could have arisen from migration of an accessory ossification centre of the adjacent cuboid (Fine 1941).

### *1.5.7 Miscellaneous Theories*

Other proposed theories include an underlying systemic metabolic or autoimmune disease (Mohiuddin et al. 2014), sequela of undiagnosed stress fracture (Mohiuddin et al. 2014), arthritis arising from dysplasia of the navicular (Viladot et al. 1987), and plastic deformation of a normal bone from mechanical overload (Simons 1930).

### *1.5.8 Osteonecrosis*

With the advent of more modern imaging techniques, Haller (San Diego, California, USA, 1988) concluded the MRI appearances of Müller-Weiss disease were consistent with osteonecrosis (Haller et al. 1988). Tan (Netherlands, 2011) provided histological evidence of osteonecrosis (Tan et al. 2011).

### *1.5.9 Link to Spanish Famine*

In 2004, Maceira and Rochera reported on the largest series of 191 feet with Müller-Weiss disease gathered from 6 centres in Spain (Maceira and Rochera 2004). Of 101 patients, 85% were manual workers from rural areas. As their birth year fitted in with the timeline of the famine brought about by the Spanish Civil War, the authors questioned whether nutritional deficiency might have interfered with normal ossification of the navicular bone.

## Delay in Ossification

They believed a combination of two factors contributed to development of Müller-Weiss disease in their patients. Firstly, they postulated that delayed ossification is a 'definite prerequisite' for the disease to occur. The navicular is the last tarsal bone to ossify. Ossification begins during the period of increased activity and mobility, at the end of the second year in girls and at the commencement of the fourth year in boys.

Delay in ossification weakens the chondral anlage of the navicular, rendering it vulnerable to plastic deformation. It can occur as part of a generalized or localized developmental disturbance. Generalized disorders that can slow or stop the ossification process in a child can be of intrinsic nature such as pluriglandular failure endocrinopathies, metabolic and malabsorption disorders or of extrinsic origin such as nutritional deficiency due to low socioeconomic status, poverty and war. Thus, Harris lines, hypoplasia of the dental enamel and metatarsal bones except of the second have been described in patients with Müller-Weiss disease.

## Overlong Second Ray

Secondly, Maceira and Rochera argued that an uneven distribution of forces is also necessary to produce compression of the lateral half of the navicular, quoting Delpech's law of physeal growth to explain overgrowth of the medial and undergrowth of the lateral half of the navicular. If compressive forces were homogenously distributed along the entire navicular, the chondral anlage would probably be able to cope and recover leaving no residual deformity except for a slight harmonic reduction of its anteroposterior dimension, as can occur in Köhler's disease.

Biomechanical conditions that can cause net lateral displacement of compressive forces acting on the navicular include congenital or acquired first ray brachymetatarsia, an overlong second ray, hypermobility of the first ray, primary subtalar joint varus and mild or underdiagnosed congenital talipes equinovarus. None of their 191 cases exhibited an index plus metatarsal formula. Most had a short first ray either because the first metatarsal itself was already short or as a result of relative shortening of the medial column due to internal rotation of the navicular in the transverse plane and retropositioning of the first tarsometatarsal (TMT1) joint relative to TMT2. A short first metatarsal does not take up compressive loads during the third rocker. Instead, the load is transferred through the second ray resulting in excessive compression of the lateral half of the navicular chondral anlage between the talar head and middle/lateral cuneiform duo (Fig. 1.1). They quoted other authors who had also noted that the first metatarsal was frequently shorter than the second. Hypermobility of the first ray has also been described in association with Müller-Weiss disease (Lafontaine et al. 1989). In a 4-year-old girl, the condition developed in one foot following traumatic epiphysiodesis of the base of the first metatarsal.

### The *Epidemic* and *Non-epidemic* Groups

In 2019, Monteagudo and Maceira reiterated the role of environmental factors in the development of Müller-Weiss disease and stated that the condition started mostly in childhood (Monteagudo and Maceira 2019). They also reaffirmed that a long second metatarsal was important for compression of the lateral navicular (Fig. 1.1).

In line with their theories, they named their first category an *epidemic* group to describe those cases believed to have resulted from the famine. Their second category consisted of a *non-epidemic* group in child athletes, who also had overlong second metatarsals. In these youngsters, they believed the disease was brought on 'by too much stress too soon' (Monteagudo and Maceira 2019). While the navicular developed normally during childhood, it deformed due to a combination of early stress from strenuous competitive sporting activities and a longer second metatarsal (See also Chap. 4 on Classification Systems).

### A Mild Form of Congenital Talipes Equinovarus

Interestingly, in 2004, Maceira and Rochera had also considered another mechanism in the pathogenesis of the *non-epidemic* form (Maceira and Rochera 2004). Among the radiological features of Müller-Weiss disease, they had described (a) parallelism of the metatarsals, especially of the first and second (b) a short first metatarsal relative to the second (c) a diarthrodial joint at the base of the first and second metatarsals giving the appearance of an elephant's foot (d) external rotation of the second tarsometatarsal (TMT) joint and (e) the axis of TMT1 facing perpendicular to the axis of the foot instead of medially (Fig. 1.2).

They had pondered upon the effect of a laterally directed force applied to the medial aspect of the first metatarsal head of an adducted forefoot with a weak navicular. An abduction force on the first metatarsal of a foot with metatarsus adductus would produce (a) abduction of the whole metatarsal palette with all metatarsals then running parallel to each other (b) friction at the base of the first metatarsal against the base of the second resulting in formation of a diarthrodial joint as seen in Müller-Weiss disease (c) external rotation of the TMT joints with TMT1 facing perpendicular to the axis of the foot instead of medially oriented (d) TMT2 externally rotated instead of facing straight ahead and (d) shortening of the first metatarsal relative to the second. Metatarsus adductus associated with some degree of heel varus constitutes a mild form of congenital talipes equinovarus (CTEV), which is easily overlooked. Based on the aforesaid mechanism, they suggested that underdiagnosed metatarsus adductus could possibly develop into Müller-Weiss disease.

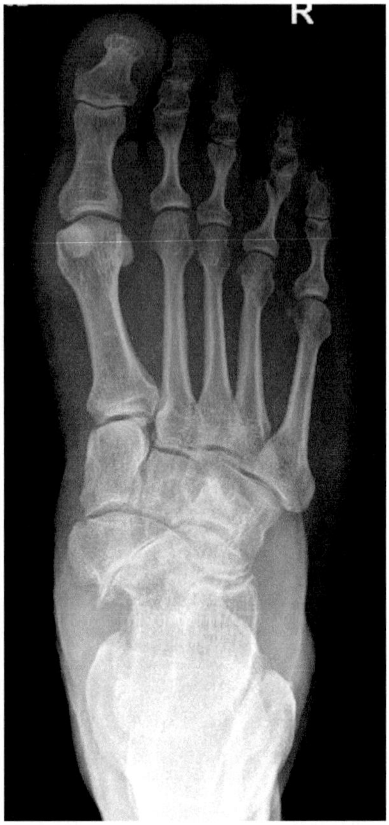


**Fig. 1.2** Dorsoplantar standing radiograph of the right foot of a 54-year-old man with late-onset Group 3B Maceira Stage V Müller-Weiss disease. Fragmentation of the lateral navicular with dorsal extrusion of the lateral fragment. Medial extrusion of the navicular pole. The talar head has shifted laterally and articulates with the lateral cuneiform, forming the talocuneiform joint characteristic of Maceira Stage V disease. Advanced osteoarthritis at the talonavicular more than at the naviculocuneiform joint. Again, note the near parallelism of the metatarsals, a short first metatarsal relative to the first, a diarthrodial joint at the base of the first metatarsal from friction against the base of the second giving the impression of an 'elephant's foot', the axis of TMT1 facing forward perpendicular to the longitudinal axis of the foot instead of medially and relative mild external rotation of TMT2 joint axis

## 1.6 The Northern Irish Experience

By contrast, Doyle et al. (2012) could not identify any environmental or socio-economic factors. Interestingly, Monteagudo and Maceira (2019) reported that most of their new cases had not suffered from nutritional or environmental stress, with an occasional new attendance from the epidemic group.

Wong-Chung et al. (2023) reported the second largest series of 95 feet, collected from the Picture and Archiving System of Northern Ireland, a population of just 1.9

million people. It is tempting to speculate that the landfall of the Spanish Armada off the West coast of Ireland may have contributed to this high incidence especially in the North-West. Genetic analysis may help elucidate. However, it would still not explain the increasing number of studies emerging from countries such as China (Zhang and Yu 2018).

Wong-Chung et al. also found predominance of an index minus metatarsal formula across all groups and subgroups, maximal in Group 3C reverse Müller-Weiss disease (Wong-Chung et al. 2023). (See also Chap. 4 on Classification Systems).

## 1.7 Timeline of Terminologies

This section tabulates the timeline of the different terminologies that came into being as a result of the various theories advanced in aetiology of the disease. The next section then seeks to clarify the confusion around nomenclature of the condition.

- 1927: Müller believed abnormal compressive forces caused the disease in an 18-year-old girl (Müller 1927). The following year, he changed his theory to a congenital cause instead.
- 1927: Weiss independently reported on the ailment and hypothesized an osteonecrotic process (Weiss 1927). The condition hence became known as Müller-Weiss disease.
- 1935: Brailsford described compression, splitting and listhesis of the navicular (Brailsford 1935a, b). To Brailsford, the dorsally displaced fragment resembled osteochondritis dissecans of the femoral condyle. He therefore named it an osteochondritis. The condition is sometimes referred to as osteochondritis and/or Brailsford's disease.
- 1937: Volk introduced the bipartite navicular (Volk 1937).
- 1981: Wiley and Brown, noting the similarity in radiographic features, used the 4 terms interchangeably implying synonymity of bipartite navicular, osteochondritis, Brailsford's disease and Müller-Weiss disease (Wiley and Brown 1981). Tanaka et al. (2006) concurred with this concept (Tanaka et al. 2006).
- Yamaguchi et al. (2016) affirmed that the bipartite navicular was a children's disease. They acknowledged that Wiley and Brown's six cases of bipartite navicular included 4 pediatric patients, aged 8 to 16 years; that Palamarchuk and Aronson (1995) equated Müller-Weiss disease with osteochondrosis in a 16-year-old female cross-country runner; and that Sharp et al. (2003) had described their 12-year-old patient as a case of osteochondritis or Brailsford's disease. Having compared the radiographs from these 3 publications, Yamaguchi et al. agreed that bipartite navicular and osteochondritis represented the same condition. However, they believed bipartite navicular and osteochondritis affected a younger age group, even though two of Wiley and Brown's patients were middle-aged adults aged 44 and 53 years (Wiley and Brown 1981). Thence, on the basis of age alone since

there were no radiographs or other details provided, they argued that the one 14-year-old boy in Doyle et al.'s series had a bipartite navicular and not Müller-Weiss disease, which is a different entity occurring in middle-aged adults with advanced arthritis (Doyle et al. 2012).

## 1.8 Standardizing Nomenclature

(a) According to Trolle's rule, the human so-called bipartite navicular does not represent true congenital partitioning. Trolle states that a true bipartition of a bone is when both fragments are equal in size and the volume of the two fragments combined would equal that of the normal bone. Trolle adds that in true partitioning, the fragments do not move away from their normal position (Trolle 1948).

In horses then, true partitioning occurs with symmetrical distribution of partitions and no separation of fragments (Zaag et al. 2016). But in humans, the lateral fragment is smaller whereas the medial fragment, which may contain an accessory navicular from the tibiale ossification centre of the first ray, is much larger (Fig. 1.1). The lateral fragment drifts dorsally and laterally whereas the medial fragment subluxes medially and plantarwards. Even if the bipartite navicular were to represent a true congenital bipartition, why should the fragments separate in utero when there is no loading of the foot? Separation could perhaps take place at a later stage, when the child starts to walk and run?

(b) In unilateral or bilateral cases, Brailsford's osteochondritis, bipartite navicular and Müller-Weiss disease have all been described with varying degrees of navicular compression and displacement of the fragments. Even Brailsford had noted that disease severity was often not equal in bilateral cases (Brailsford 1939). While the more severely affected foot exhibited splitting of the navicular with marked separation of the two fragments, the contralateral side would demonstrate less extensive changes 'such as mere compression of the plastic outer third of the navicular' with no splitting. Brailsford also described what we nowadays know to be end-stage Maceira Stage V disease in which 'ultimately these cuneiform surfaces may even articulate with the head of the astragalus'. Maceira and Rochera referred to the latter as the talocuneiform articulation, while more contemporary authors have used the terms 'talocuneiform pseudarthrosis' or 'talocuneiform neoarticulation' (Kani et al. 2016; Joseph et al. 2021).

Recent literature also contains examples of bilateral disease with severe Stage V on one side and mild affection at the other foot. Figure 1.3 illustrates such an example of a woman born around the same time as Brailsford and Volk described osteochondritis and the bipartite navicular, respectively. She first presented in 2010 at the age of 64 years and has not required surgery to either foot. By contemporary standards, her right foot would be designated as a Maceira Stage V Müller-Weiss disease whereas Brailsford would have labelled it as an osteochondritis and Volk, Wiley and Brown as a bipartite navicular. Her left foot showed lesser degrees of compression and degeneration.

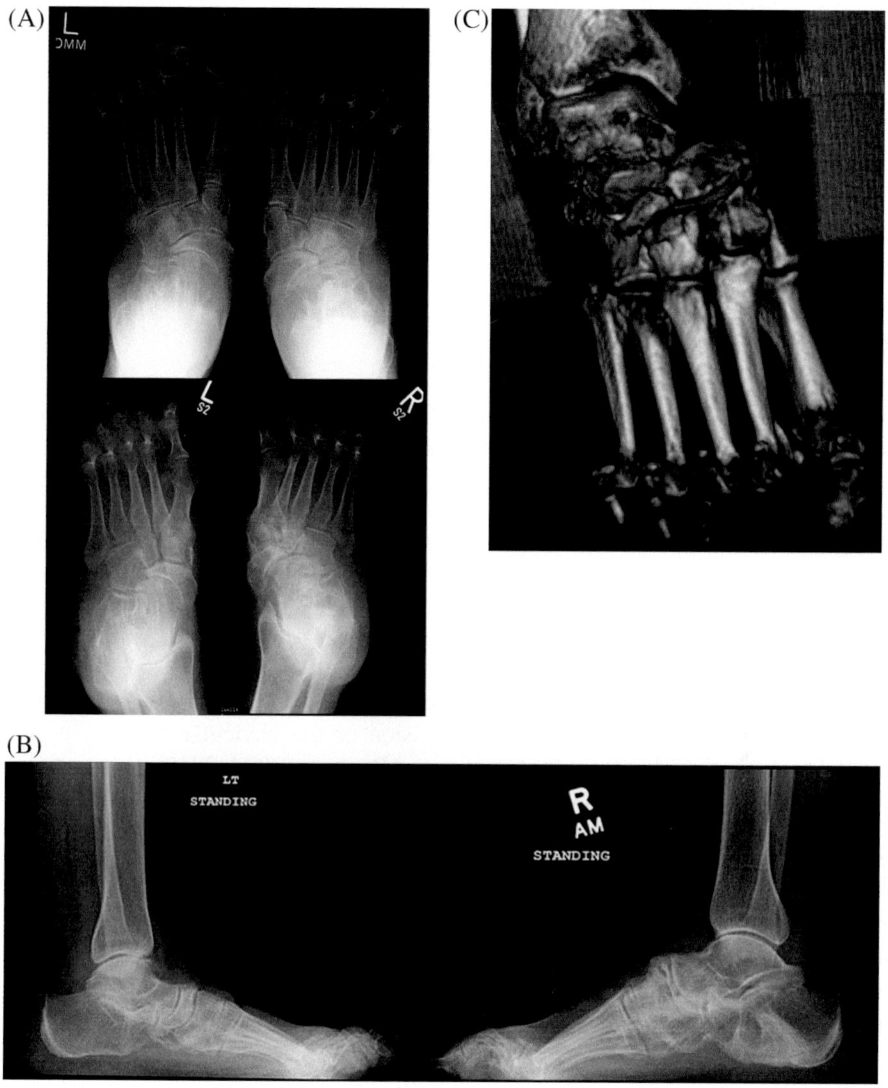


**Fig. 1.3** Dorsoplantar standing and medial oblique radiographs (A) of both feet of a 74-year-old woman demonstrating end-stage disease on the right side. Mild navicular compression and perinavicular degenerative changes. (B) Note the Harris line in the distal right tibia and areas of bone necrosis in the right calcaneum on arch views. (C) 3D-CT volume rendering image shows marked medial talonavicular subluxation and dorsally displaced navicular fragment articulating with corresponding facet on the dorsum of the lateral cuneiform

The foregoing points support the views of the other authors who believe that the terms Brailsford's disease, osteochondritis, bipartite navicular and Müller-Weiss disease refer to one and the same condition. The radiographic appearances in the more severe forms of bipartite navicular and Brailsford's osteochondritis are identical to Stage V of Maceira's classification of Müller-Weiss disease. When fragmentation of the lateral navicular has taken place, varying degrees of separation of the two fragments can occur. Those with wide separation and displacement of the fragments came to be labelled as a bipartite navicular by some and as an osteochondritis by others. Both the terms Brailsford's disease and Müller-Weiss disease include cases with and without fragmentation. The bipartite navicular only includes instances where fragmentation has occurred and usually with a wide degree of separation of the fragments.

### *1.8.1 Evolution*

Knowledge of its evolution would answer the numerous unknowns about the condition. Maceira and Rochera stated that, although they had observed increasing compression and degeneration in the same foot, they had not encountered a case in which the stage of the disease changed. They therefore argued that, except for the Müller-Weissoid feet, Müller-Weiss changes began in childhood and remained asymptomatic until late adulthood, as did Wiley and Brown. Wong-Chung et al. (2023) grouped 95 feet into early-onset and late-onset disease. None of their early-onset disease had required surgery. They also thought it conceivable that the disease developed in childhood and became manifest in adulthood.

The first question then is the age at which disease starts. Contemporary theories favor an asymmetrical mechanical compression of the navicular by an overlong second metatarsal as theorized by Maceira and Rochera (2004, 2019), substantiated by Wong-Chung et al. (2023) in 2023 and observed as far back as 1935 by Brailsford (1939). In addition, Maceira and Monteagudo stipulate that the navicular anlage must also have been weakened by delay in ossification from either intrinsic or extrinsic factors.

For the sake of discussion, supposing there may be a congenital element of partitioning, the fragments should not separate in utero where there is no loading on the foot. Loading would only begin when the child starts to walk at the age of 12 months or run between 18 and 24 months old.

The navicular begins ossification at between 18 to 24 months in girls and between 30 to 36 months in boys. To define when normality changes to pathology, the ideal longitudinal study should include radiographs from around or predating these age groups. However, practically speaking, such studies are not feasible, because it is not known which feet will develop Müller-Weiss disease. Nor is it known why some Morton's type feet develop Müller-Weiss changes as a consequence of a short first ray and others do not.

The next question is what happens to the lateral navicular fragment, once fragmentation has occurred. Initially undisplaced, does it progress to full displacement to reach Maceira end-stage V disease? Fig. 1.4 illustrates a 12-year-old girl with bilateral disease characterized by fragmentation at the lateral navicular and marked medial talonavicular subluxation. CT scan confirms that the lateral navicular fragment is slightly displaced laterally with no dorsal displacement. It remains undisplaced 11 years later and the woman is still asymptomatic at the age of 33 years old.

As previously mentioned, in the largest series worldwide, Maceira and Rochera did not come across any case in which the stage of the disease had changed. Similarly, in the second largest series, Wong-Chung et al. did not encounter any case in which the grouping had changed.

What this means is that affected feet present, each at its own different stage or belonging to a particular group. That stage or group does not tend to change with time. There is no case series of a lateral navicular fragment progressing from an undisplaced position to marked dorsal and lateral displacement as with a bipartite navicular or in Stage V on Maceira's classification of Müller-Weiss disease. Researchers can hence only infer the evolution of the disease from a spectrum of the different snapshots of the way the disease presents. This should be borne in mind when considering the pathomechanics of the condition (See Chap. 4 on Classifications systems).

**Concluding Remarks**

Our predecessors did remarkably well to bring this condition to attention. In particular, Brailsford is to be credited for his detailed radiographic description of the disease, with little else to add almost nine decades later.

Bipartite navicular has been posited as a cause of Müller-Weiss disease (Yamaguchi et al. 2016). Doubt exists regarding true congenital partitioning of the human navicular. This author believes that the terms Brailsford's osteochondritis, bipartite navicular and Müller-Weiss disease all refer to the same condition, which can present with varying degrees of navicular compression, fragmentation and fragment separation. When fragmentation occurs, the fragments may be juxtaposed initially. Although there are no longitudinal studies to prove that undisplaced fragmentation of the lateral navicular progresses to full-blown separation, it is believed that separation ensues with the lateral fragment displacing laterally and dorsally, while the medial fragment subluxes medially and plantarwards. When separation is great enough, the talar head articulates directly with the lateral cuneiform, forming the talocuneiform articulation, which marks Stage V on Maceira's classification of Müller-Weiss disease. This Author posits that the severe forms of bipartite navicular and Brailsford's osteochondritis represent Stage V Müller-Weiss disease on Maceira's classification. This end-stage disease with marked separation of the fragments became designated as a bipartite navicular by some and Brailsford's osteochondritis by others. While the term bipartite navicular is restricted to those feet with splitting of the navicular whatever the degree of separation of fragments, the terms Brailsford's disease and Müller-Weiss disease encompass those with and without fragmentation.

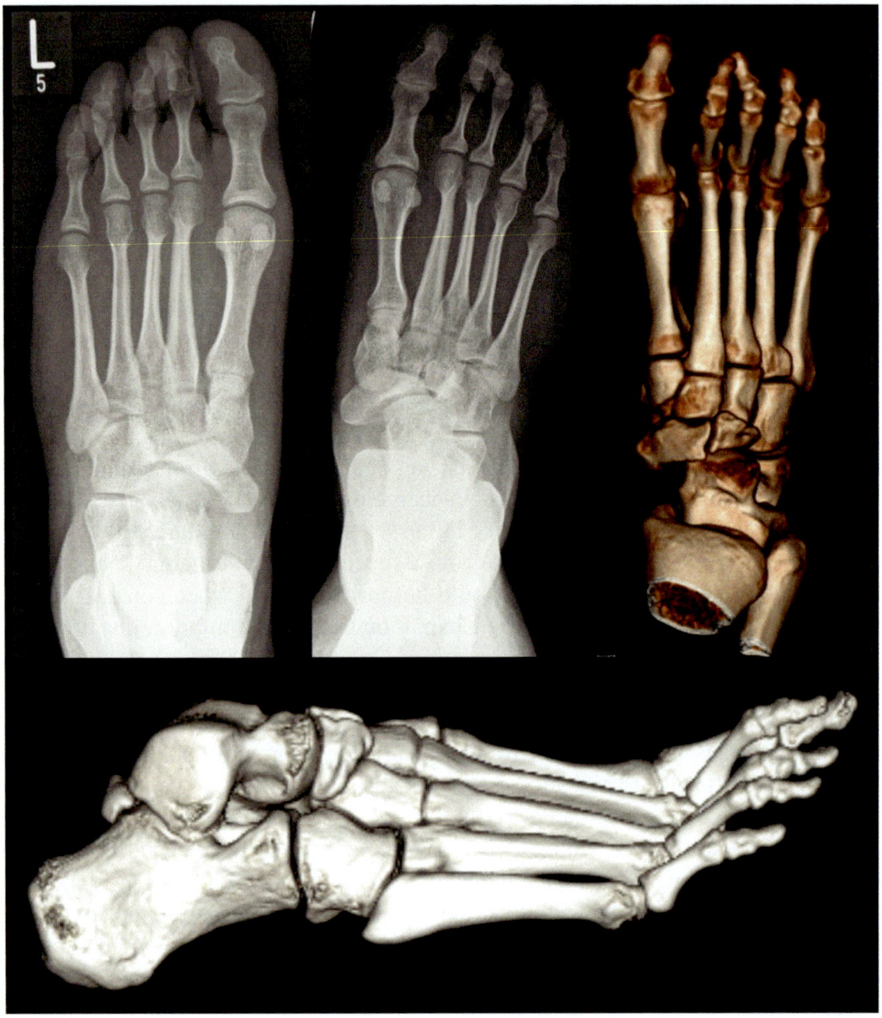


**Fig. 1.4** Dorsoplantar standing radiographs of a 12-year-old girl with bilateral early-onset Müller-Weiss disease. Fragmentation at the lateral navicular and marked medial talonavicular subluxation. CT scan demonstrates only slight lateral displacement of the lateral navicular fragment with no dorsal displacement as yet. It is much smaller than the medial fragment

Therefore, for the sake of uniformity, the term osteochondritis, Brailsford disease and bipartite navicular will not be used throughout the remainder of this book, except in passing and in Chap. 12 where surgery was believed to have been performed for these diagnoses.

Current consensus on aetiology of Müller-Weiss disease is of a lateral shift in compression forces acting upon the navicular brought about by a long second metatarsal or insufficiency of the first ray. Another yet unidentified factor must predispose the navicular to deform under eccentric compression stress in some cases, since not all naviculars of Morton's type feet undergo deformation.

## References


Brailsford JF. Osteochondritis. Br J Radiol. 1935a;NS8:87–134.

Brailsford JF. Osteochondritis. In: London J, Churchill A, editors. The radiology of bones and joints, 2nd ed.; 1935b.

Brailsford JF. Osteochondritis of the adult tarsal navicular. J Bone Joint Surg. 1939;21(1):111–20.

Brailsford JF. Osteochondritis. In: London J, Churchill A, editors. The radiology of bones and joints, 5th ed.; 1953.

Chujo T, Nakasa T, Ikuta Y, Kawabata S, Adachi N. Talonavicular arthrodesis using a screw and compression staple in a patient with bipartite navicular bone: a case report. Cureus. 2023;15(8):e43122. https://doi.org/10.7759/cureus.43122.

Coughlin MJ. Sesamoid and accessory bones of the foot. In: Coughlin MJ, Mann RA, Saltman CL, editors. Surgery of the foot and ankle. bipartite navicular, vol. 10, 8th ed. Philadelphia, PA: Mosby Elsevier; 2007. p. 595–6.

De Fine LE. On bipartite os naviculare pedis. Acta Radiol. 1941;22:377–82.

Doyle T, Napier RJ, Wong-Chung J. Recognition and management of Müller-Weiss disease. Foot Ankle Int. 2012;33(4):275–81. https://doi.org/10.3113/FAI.2012.0275.

Haller J, Sartoris DJ, Resnick D, Pathria MN, Berthoty D, Howard B, Nordstrom D. Spontaneous osteonecrosis of the tarsal navicular in adults: imaging findings. AJR Am J Roentgenol. 1988;151:355–8. https://doi.org/10.2214/ajr.151.2.355.

Hatoff A. Bipartite navicular bone as a cause of flatfoot. AMA Am J Dis Child. 1950;80(6):991–2. https://doi.org/10.1001/archpedi.1950.04040021006013.

Joseph VM, Lynser D, Khan AY, Daniala C. Mueller Weiss syndrome, a less elucidated and unusual cause of midfoot pain: a case report. Indian J Musculoskelet Radiol. 2021;3(2):94–7. https://doi.org/10.25259/IJMSR_47_2020

Kani KK, Mulcahy H, Chew FS. Case 228: Mueller-Weiss disease. Radiology. 2016;279:317–21. https://doi.org/10.1148/radiol.2016132280.

Lafontaine M, Charlier PH, Hardy D, Delince P. Hypermobilité du premier rayon associée à une ostéonécrose-fracture du scaphoïde tarsien [Hypermobility of the first ray associated with osteonecrosis-fracture of the tarsal navicular bone]. Acta Orthop Belg. 1989;55(4):565–71.

Maceira E, Rochera R. Müller-Weiss disease: clinical and biomechanical features. Foot Ankle Clin. 2004;9(1):105–25. https://doi.org/10.1016/s1083-7515(03)00153-0.

Mau H. Zur kenntnis des naviculare bipartitum pedis. Z Orthop. 1960;93:404.

Mohiuddin T, Jennison T, Damany D. Müller–Weiss disease. Review of current knowledge. Foot Ankle Surg. 2014;20(2):79–84. https://doi.org/10.1016/j.fas.2013.11.001

Monteagudo M, Maceira E. Management of Müller-Weiss disease. Foot Ankle Clin. 2019;24(1):89–105. https://doi.org/10.1016/j.fcl.2018.09.006.

Müller W. Über eine eigenartige doppelseitige veränderung des os naviculare beim Erwachsenen [On an odd double-sided change of the tarsal navicular]. Deutsche Zeitschrift Für Chirurgie Leipzig. 1927;201:84–7.

Palamarchuk HJ, Aronson SM. Osteochondrosis of the tarsal navicular in a female high school distance runner. J Am Podiatr Med Assoc. 1995;85(4):226–9. https://doi.org/10.7547/87507315-85-4-226.

Rijkenhuizen ABM, Németh F, Dik KJ, Goedegebuure SA. The arterial supply of the navicular bone in the normal horse. Equine Vet J. 1989;21:399–404.

Sarrafian SK. Osteology. In: Kelikian AS editor. Sarrafian's anatomy of the foot and ankle, vol. 2, 3rd ed. Philadelphia, PA: Lippincott, Williams & Wilkins; 2011. p. 116.

Sharp RJ, Calder JD, Saxby TS. Osteochondritis of the navicular: a case report. Foot Ankle Int. 2003;24(6):509–13. https://doi.org/10.1177/107110070302400611.

Shawdon A, Kiss ZS, Fuller P. The bipartite tarsal navicular bone: radiographic and computed tomography findings. Australas Radiol. 1995;39(2):192–4. https://doi.org/10.1111/j.1440-1673.1995.tb00271.x.

Simons B. Über osteopathia deformans des os naviculare pedis [On osteopathia deformans of the tarsal navicular]. Z Orthop Chir. 1930;52:564–8.

Tan A, Smulders YCMM, Zöphel OT. Use of remodeled femoral head allograft for tarsal reconstruction in the treatment of Müller-Weiss disease. J Foot Ankle Surg. 2011;50(6):721–6. https://doi.org/10.1053/j.jfas.2011.04.043.

Tanaka Y, Takakura Y, Omokawa S, Kumai T, Sugimoto K. Crank-shaped arthrodesis for a flatfoot with a bipartite navicular: a case report. Foot Ankle Int. 2006;27(9):734–7. https://doi.org/10.1177/107110070602700914.

Torg JS, Pavlov H, Cooley LH, Bryant MH, Arnoczky SP, Bergfeld J, Hunter LY. Stress fractures of the tarsal navicular. A retrospective review of twenty-one cases. J Bone Joint Surg [Am]. 1982;64(5):700–12.

Trolle D. Accessory bones of the human foot. In: A radiological, histoembryological, comparative anatomical and genetic study. Copenhagen, Munksgaard; 1948. pp. 150–1.

Van der Zaag EJ, Weerts EAWS, Van den Belt AJM, Back W. Clinicopathological findings in horses with a bi- or tripartite navicular bone. BMC Vet Res. 2016;12–74. https://doi.org/10.1186/s12917-016-0698-4

Viladot A, Rochera R, Viladot A Jr. Necrosis of the navicular bone. Bull Hosp Jt Dis Orthop Inst. 1987;47(2):285–93.

Volk C. Zwei fälle von os naviculare pedis bipartitum. Z Orthop Ihre Grenzgeb. 1937;66:396–403.

Weiss K. Über die "malazie" des os naviculare pedis [On the malacia of the tarsal navicular]. Fortschr Geb Rontgenstr. 1927;45:63–7.

Wiley JJ, Brown DE. The bipartite tarsal scaphoid. J Bone Joint Surg. 1981;63B(4):583–6.

Wong-Chung J, Walls A, Lynch-Wong M, Cassidy R, McKenna R, Wilson A, Stephens M. Towards understanding Müller-Weiss disease from an analysis of 95 cases. Foot Ankle Surg. 2023;29(5):401–11. https://doi.org/10.1016/j.fas.2023.05.004.

Yamaguchi S, Niki H, Akagi R, Yamamoto Y, Sasho T. Failure of internal fixation for painful bipartite navicular in two adolescent soccer players: a report of two cases. J Foot Ankle Surg. 2016;55(6):1323–6. https://doi.org/10.1053/j.jfas.2016.01.015.

Zhang M-Z, Yu G. Surgical treatment for Müller-Weiss disease. Foot & Ankle Orthop. 2018;3(3). https://doi.org/10.1177/2473011418S00536

Zimmer EA. Krankheiten, verletzungen und varietaten des os naviculare pedis. Arch Orthop Unfall Chir. 1938;38:396–411.

# Chapter 2
# Clinical Features

**Abstract** A relatively rare condition, Müller-Weiss disease is being increasingly recognized worldwide through greater awareness. Frequently bilateral, it affects females predominantly. It has been reported in all 5 continents. The first biggest study came from Spain. With a noticeable dearth of literature from the Americas, large series have recently emerged from Northern Ireland, Thailand and China. Sometimes discovered as an incidental finding, many patients often give a long-standing history of spontaneous onset of symptoms before seeking medical attention. Degree of deformity does not correlate with severity of symptoms. When evaluating peekaboo sign for subtle hindfoot varus, it is important to view the heels at ankle level and not from an elevated height at knee level. Palpate each perinavicular joint for tenderness in preparation for selection of which joints to fuse if arthrodesis surgery is required. Depending on stage of the disease, the medial arch may be elevated, normal or flattened. Heel varus is not always the rule. When the arch is flat and the heel is in varus, the term 'paradoxical pes planus varus' may then be correctly applied. In the differential diagnosis of Müller-Weiss disease, Köhler's disease and navicular stress fractures demonstrate different clinical and radiographic characteristics.

**Keywords** Müller-Weiss disease · Navicular · Paradoxical pes planus varus · Peekaboo sign · Perinavicular joints · Nutritional deficiency

## Introduction

First described in Europe, with a particularly high incidence in Spain, Müller-Weiss disease is being increasingly reported worldwide through greater awareness and better recognition. Of insidious onset, it is believed to start in childhood but becomes manifest mostly during the fifth decade of life. Other than tenderness and some swelling on palpation, physical examination may reveal little else especially in the way of deformity. The prominence at the medial aspect of the foot is caused not by the talar head as in progressive collapsing foot deformity, but by a medially displaced navicular tuberosity, giving the impression of a flatfoot. The medial arch itself may be high or low or within normal range.

© The Author(s), under exclusive license to Springer Nature Switzerland AG 2024

J. Wong-Chung, *Comprehensive Guide to Müller-Weiss Disease*,
https://doi.org/10.1007/978-3-031-66644-5_2

The term 'paradoxical pes planus varus' has been coined to characterize heel varus with associated flatfoot as hallmark deformities of the disease.

This Chapter goes through the steps of history-taking and a systematic orthopaedic physical examination consisting of inspection, palpation and movements. In particular, it focuses on assessment of hindfoot position by inspection for peekaboo sign and palpation for spatial orientation of the heel. It questions the notion of obligatory heel varus in Müller-Weiss disease.

## 2.1 Epidemiology

### *2.1.1 Incidence*

Müller-Weiss disease is classified as a rare disease (Mueller-Weiss Disease 2022). It was not widely known even among the medical community (Doyle et al. 2012; Maceira and Rochera 2004), until the public came to hear all about it in May 2022 when its diagnosis was announced in contemporary tennis champion, Rafael Nadal Parera of Manacor, Spain (Roy 2022). Rafa was diagnosed with the disease in 2005 and has had symptoms since his late teens at the beginning of his career. He probably falls into the *non-epidemic* category of child athletes, subjected to "too much too soon", as described by his fellow countrymen Monteagudo and Maceira (Monteagudo and Maceira 2019). He has put off surgery, relying purely on pain management. Despite his painful foot, he has won 92 Association of Tennis Professionals (ATP) singles titles, including 22 Grand Slam men's singles and 36 ATP Tour Masters 1000 titles to date.

### *2.1.2 Age*

Mean age at diagnosis, 47.6 $\pm$ 14.4 (range, 13–91) years (Maceira and Rochera 2004).

### *2.1.3 Sex Distribution*

It occurs predominantly in females. Of the 191 feet reported by Maceira and Rochera, 73% were women (Maceira and Rochera 2004). In 1939, all 9 cases of Brailsford were women (Brailsford 1939) and in 2023, 55% of Wong-Chung et al.'s 67 patients were female (Wong-Chung et al. 2023).

### 2.1.4 Laterality

Frequently bilateral (Doyle et al. 2012). All 9 cases of Brailsford were bilateral in 1939 (Brailsford 1939) and 42% of Wong-Chung et al.'s cases were bilateral in 2023 (Wong-Chung et al. 2023).

### 2.1.5 Heredity

According to the National Organization for Rare Diseases (NORD), there is no evidence of a genetic cause and it does not tend to run in families (Mueller-Weiss Disease 2022). Among the 95 feet in the series of Wong-Chung et al., there were 2 brothers who presented with bilateral reverse Müller-Weiss disease in their mid-50's (Wong-Chung et al. 2023). Both have proceeded to corrective surgery. None of the other patients were closely related. In one 76-year-old woman with bilateral disease, DNA testing from Ancestry.com revealed she was 95% Irish with no Spanish connection.

### 2.1.6 Geographical Distribution

Maceira and Rochera (Spain, 2004) opined that the dearth of literature from North America compared to Europe suggested predisposing environmental and nutritional factors were at play (Maceira and Rochera 2004). More recently, some of the largest surgical series have emanated from China (Zhang and Yu 2017, 2018; Yuan et al. 2019). Angthong et al. (Thailand, 2023) stated that 0.6% of patients presenting at his foot and ankle clinic suffer from Müller-Weiss disease (Angthong et al. 2023).

Chiavegatti et al. (2018) presented the earliest known ancient case of Müller-Weiss disease in a male believed to have lived 2300 years ago. His skeleton was discovered in a sarcophagus during an archaeological project undertaken jointly by the Museu Egipci de Barcelona, Spain and the Eberhard Karls Universtat, Tübingen, Germany at the necropolis of Sharuna in Middle Egypt, 200 km south of El Cairo on the east bank of the river Nile. Judging by its housing, the sarcophagus dated from the end of the Late period (380 BC) to the beginning of the Hellenistic period (150 BC) during the Ptolemaic dynasty. Age at time of death was estimated at between 21 and 30 years old.

The skeleton exhibited evidence of marked compression of the lateral part of both navicular bones with advanced degenerative changes at the talonavicular joints and prominent dorsal osteophytes at the talar neck. Also noted elsewhere were dental attrition and avascular necrosis with associated degenerative changes at the right humeral head. The authors estimated the disease to have been at Stage I or II. Besides Stage I being a diagnosis that is made by MRI, it would have been impossible to evaluate disease stage without weight-bearing radiographs. The photograph provided shows a left talus with its lateral talar process facing laterally. The navicular tuberosity, which is normally situated medially, has been positioned so that it also faces laterally. This probably represents either a malrotation of the navicular in the photograph or a mismatch of right and left sides of talus and navicular.

From Egypt in more recent years, Ahmed et al. (Qalyubia, Egypt, 2019) has published a case series of 13 feet in 7 adolescents with early-onset Müller-Weiss disease (Ahmed et al. 2019). The pattern of disease in their young patients may differ from those of Wong-Chung et al. in Northern Ireland (Wong-Chung et al. 2023). (See Chap. 4 on Classification Systems).

Eloundou et al. (Cameroon, 2020) reported on a 35-year-old amateur tennis player whom they believed to be the only case of Müller-Weiss disease to have been described in sub-Saharan Africa (Eloundou et al. 2020). The condition was graded at Maceira Stage IV. However, MRI scan demonstrated a talo-cuneiform articulation, making it a Stage V disease. No plain radiographs are available and from the MR images provided, it is not possible to assess which group it belongs to. The case was treated by arthrodesis, of which no further details are available.

### 2.1.7 *Body Mass Index*

Fornaciari et al. (2014) reported a mean BMI of 29.6 kg/m$^2$ in their 10 patients while BMI averaged 27 kg/m$^2$ in the 6 patients of Hetsroni et al. (2007).

## 2.2 Presenting Symptoms

Patients commonly give a long-standing history of spontaneous onset of pain on the dorsum of the midfoot ± hindfoot. Minor trauma may precipitate symptoms in 10% of cases. Some complain of functional lateral ankle instability with referred pain around the peroneal tendons (Monteagudo and Maceira 2019).

Symptoms may be well tolerated for years. Doyle et al. quoted a mean duration of symptoms of 5.2 years in 4 men and 8 women (Doyle et al. 2012). De Fine Licht remarked that the condition can remain asymptomatic for most yet prove crippling in others by their second or third decade (Fine 1941).

### 2.2.1 *Incidentaloma*

Müller-Weiss disease is sometimes detected as an incidental finding on radiography obtained for other reason, commonly trauma (Ahmed et al. 2019; Bartolotta et al. 2014).

Bartolotta et al. (NY, 2014) reported on a 32-year-old healthy woman who presented with pain over the dorsum of the first metatarsal head following a minor stumble (Bartolotta et al. 2014). She had no foot symptoms prior to the fall. Plain radiographs demonstrated a 'comma-shaped' navicular with compression and sclerosis of its lateral aspect, which the authors regarded as the hallmark radiographic signs of Müller-Weiss disease. Lateral shift of the talar head and a decreased Kite's angle were deemed indicative of hindfoot varus.

Pain at the first metatarsal subsided with physical therapy. Two years later, she re-attended with chronic pain and intermittent swelling centered around the navicular. Repeat radiographs showed increasing sclerosis with a recent sagittal cleft running from distal dorsal to proximal plantar and slight dorsal extrusion of the lateral fragment. MRI revealed bone marrow oedema in the dorsolateral aspect of the navicular.

There was no further mention of treatment, since the theme of the publication was that radiological signs predated development of symptoms in their patient.

## 2.3 Clinical Examination

### *2.3.1 Look*

Observe the patient walking for any gait abnormality. During the erect examination, either from in front or from behind, the patient stands with both feet at shoulder width. For a proper assessment of heel position, it is imperative that the medial borders of both feet should be parallel. Looking from the front, the toes point towards the examiner (Figs. 2.1, 2.2 and 2.3).

Front: Note that the prominence at the medial side of the foot is formed by the navicular tuberosity, giving the false impression of a collapsed medial arch (Fig. 2.1E-F). It is not due to the talar head as in progressive collapsing foot deformity (PCFD). In fact, the talar head lies in the midline of the foot and points laterally and plantarwards, and not medially (Fig. 2.1G).

Arch: Depending upon Maceira stage of the disease, the medial longitudinal arch can be (i) normal (ii) high or (iii) low.

Heel position: When the talar head points medially as in PCFD, the calcaneus shifts laterally. Maceira and Rochera reasoned that the corollary also applies. Therefore, according to them, when the talar head points laterally as in Müller-Weiss disease, the heel should automatically move into varus. They stated that all of their 191 cases had heel varus. They concluded that the heel must always be in varus in Müller-Weiss disease. They coined the term "paradoxical pes planus varus", as a result of which, heel varus has since been regarded as a hallmark deformity of Müller-Weiss disease.

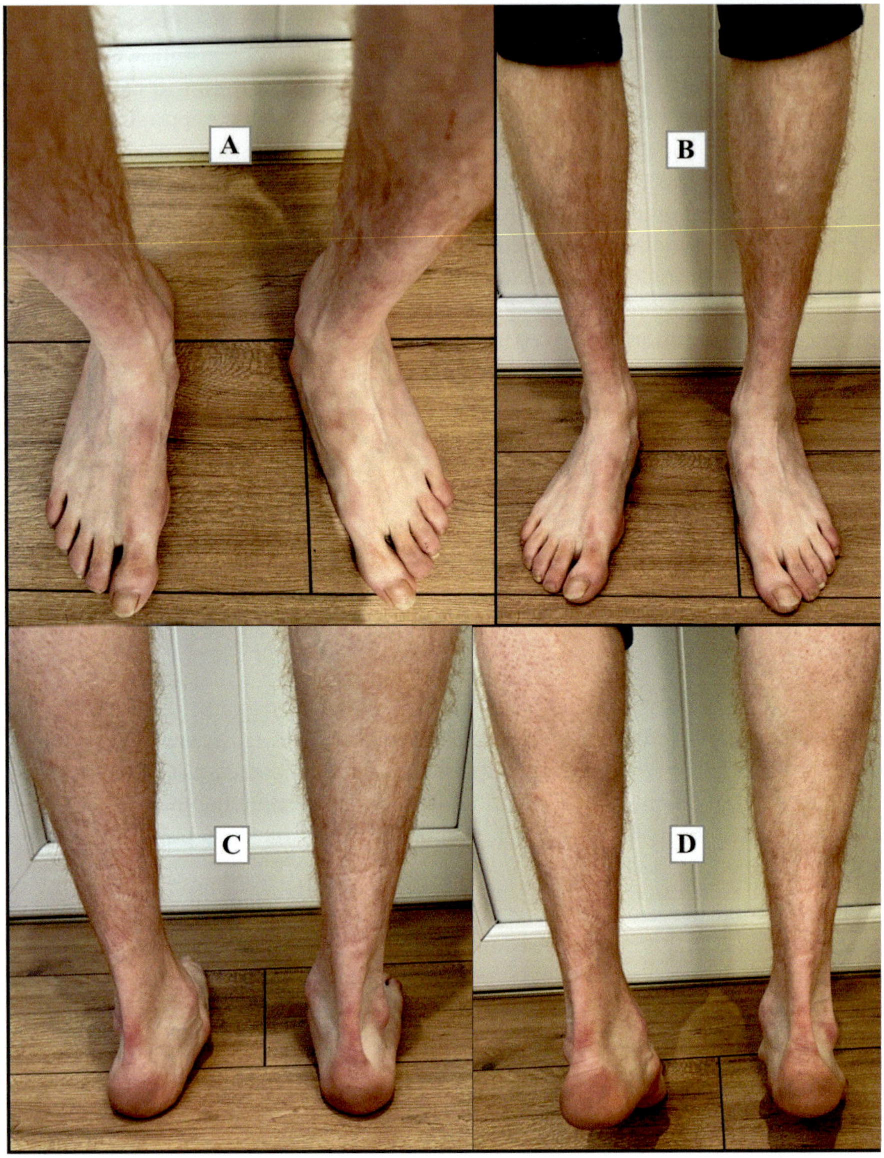


But is heel varus really mandatory for the diagnosis of Müller-Weiss disease? Fig. 2.1 illustrates a case in which the heels are in valgus whereas Fig. 2.2 demonstrates an example with the heels in varus. (See also Sects. 3.7 and 3.8 in Chap. 3 on Radiographic Features).

Close analysis of the illustrations provided by Maceira and Rochera (2004) in 2004 and again in 2019 by Monteagudo and Maceira (Monteagudo and Maceira 2019) reveals that heels were deemed clinically in varus, looking downwards from

◄**Fig. 2.1** A not-so 'paradoxical pes planus varus.' Clinical photographs of a 29-year-old man with bilateral Müller-Weiss disease, more marked on the left side (published with patient's consent). (A) Viewed from above, the medial aspects of both heels are visible. Note the degree of midfoot abduction of the left foot. (B) Frontal view at ankle level. The patient stands with feet at shoulder width, the medial border of both feet parallel and the toes pointing towards the examiner. Peekaboo sign is negative. (C) Rear view. Again, the patient stands with feet at shoulder width, the medial border of both feet parallel and the toes pointing straight ahead. Marked valgus offset of the left and mild valgus offset of the right heel. (D) Both heels do not varize and both arches do not correct completely when standing on tiptoes. (E, F) Medial view. Prominence at the medial arch is formed by a prominent navicular tuberosity and not by the talar head as in progressive collapsing deformity. (G) In fact, the talar head lies laterally towards the centre of the foot as shown on dorsoplantar standing radiograph. Also note the cortical hypertrophy of an overlong second metatarsal, striking parallelism of the metatarsals and the hallucal sesamoids sitting in "too pretty" position. (H) Medial oblique radiograph shows marked compression of the lateral portion of the navicular. (I) Lateral standing radiograph of the left ankle and foot demonstrates dorsal extrusion of the lateral navicular fragment and mild sagging at the naviculocuneiform joint. (J, K) Hindfoot alignment radiographs obtained with the tibia in line with the second toe confirm marked valgus offset of the left heel and mild valgus of the right heel

above knee level. From an elevated eye level, even normal heels will demonstrate an apparent positive 'peekaboo sign' (Fig. 2.3A–C) (Manoli et al. 1993; Manoli and Graham 2005). In both the 2004 and 2019 illustrations, direct frontal and rear photographs clearly show negative 'peekaboo sign' and physiological heel valgus, respectively.

Maceira and Rochera (2004) further remarked that heel varus can be subtle and appreciable only by palpation. In 2019, Monteagudo and Maceira added that palpation may only detect heel varus during heel rise and subtalar movement. This method of evaluating heel position will yield further false positive heel varus, because in the presence of a flexible subtalar joint, heels normally move into varus when standing on tip toes due to the action of the posterior tibial tendon (Fig. 2.3D). By visually assessing peekaboo sign from an elevated bird's-eye view and heel varus by palpation when standing on tip toes, all heels will appear in varus. This calls into question whether all cases of Müller-Weiss disease truly had obligatory heel varus.

Frigg et al. had demonstrated less than 50% correlation between visual assessment and radiographic hindfoot alignment (Frigg et al. 2010). A better clinical evaluation of heel position can be obtained using a combination of inspection and palpation, by holding the heel locked in eversion in the palm of the examiner's hand with the patient supine or sitting, and visualizing its position in space, be it varus, neutral or valgus.

### 2.3.2 *Feel*

Palpate each of the perinavicular (talonavicular, subtalar, calcaneocuboid and naviculocuneiform) joints for tenderness to assist decision-making on selection of joints to arthrodese.

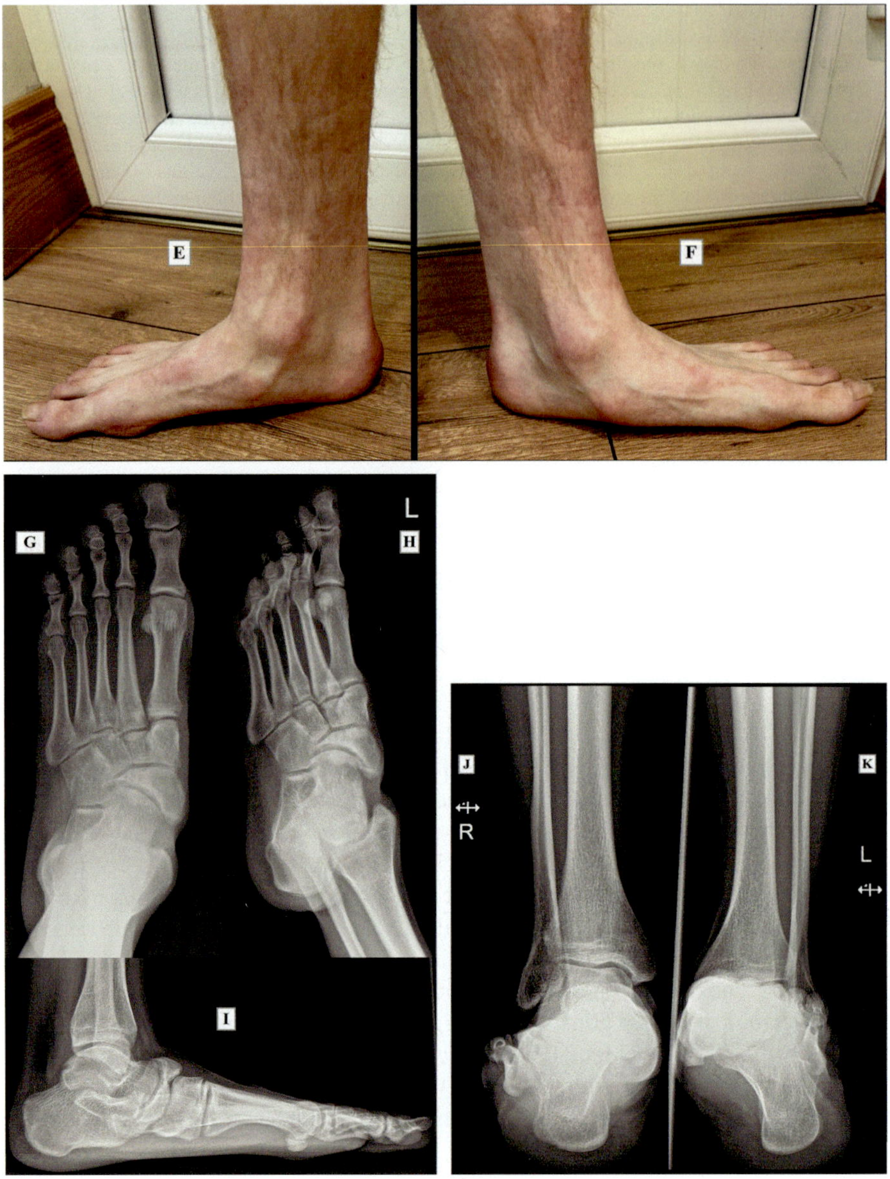


Fig. 2.1 (continued)

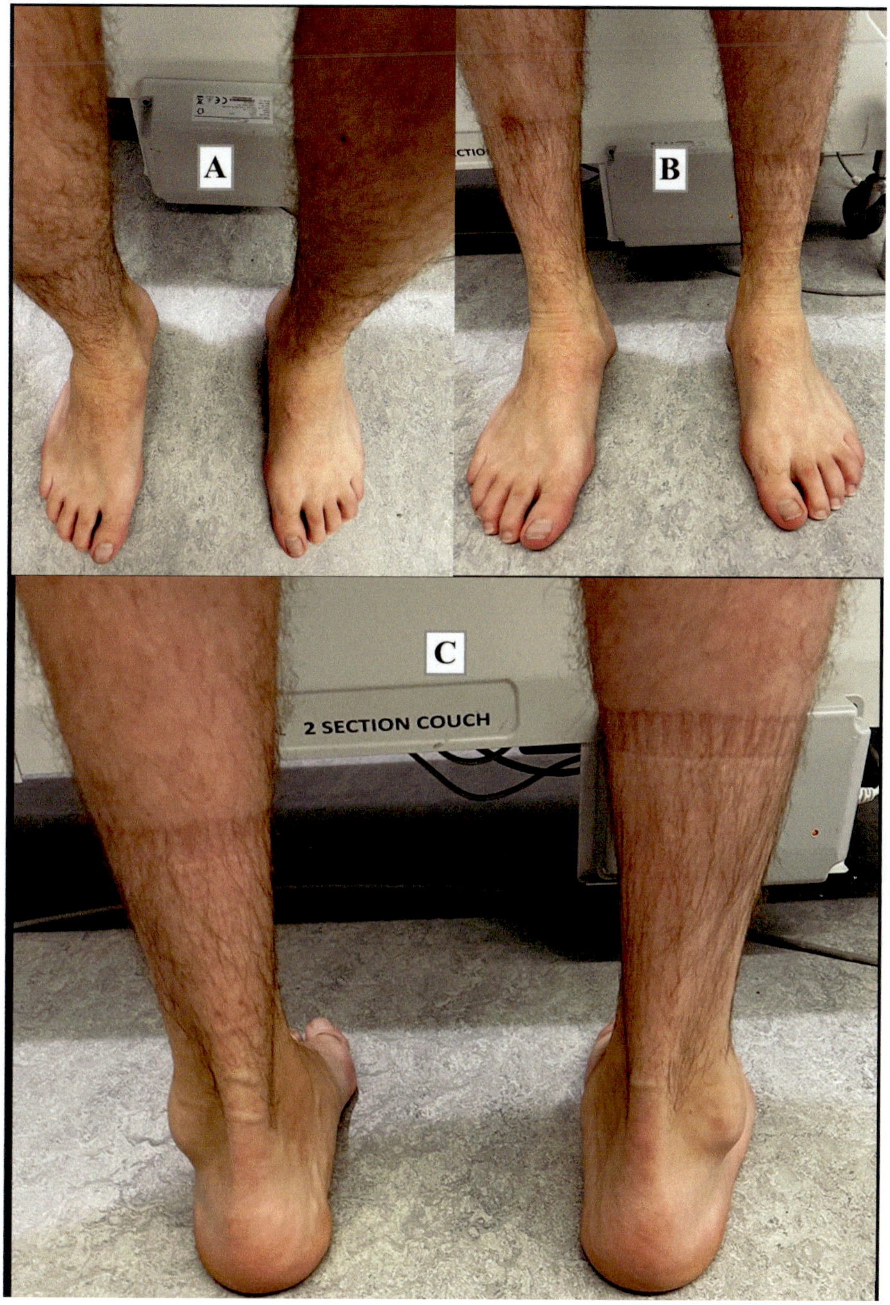
A
B
C
2 SECTION COUCH

◀**Fig. 2.2** True heel varus. Clinical photographs of a 20-year-old man with bilateral Müller-Weiss disease (published with patient's consent). (A) Viewed from above, the medial aspects of both heels are visible. (B) Viewed from in front at ankle level, true peekaboo signs can now be said to be positive as (C) viewed from behind, both heels are in varus. (D, E) Prominences at medial arch are formed by the navicular tuberosities and not the talar heads, which lie laterally in the centre of the foot as shown on (F, G) dorsoplantar standing radiographs of both feet. Tenting of skin overlying prominent navicular tuberosities. Fragmentation of the lateral navicular and medial extrusion of its medial pole bilaterally. (H) Dorsal extrusion of the lateral navicular fragment with normal Méary's angle on the left. (I) Right Maceira Stage II with mild apex dorsal arch. Sagittal clefts are seen running from distal dorsal to proximal plantar

Swelling and tenderness is normally present at the dorsomedial aspect of the midfoot. The anterior and plantar aspect of the heel is prominent from the calcaneocuboid joint. The heel is prominent posteriorly due to rearfoot equinus (Maceira and Rochera 2004) and relative advancement of the tibia in relation to the tarsal joints (Mohiuddin et al. 2014).

### 2.3.3 *Move*

Subtalar and mid-tarsal movements are usually reduced.

## 2.4 Other Signs and Symptoms

Toes are characteristically parallel to each other. Hallux valgus is uncommon in association with Müller-Weiss disease.

"Pes planus varus" forces the tibia into external rotation with resultant retropositioning of the fibula, whereas the leg is usually internally rotated in PCFD. Theoretically, this alters knee biomechanics and patellar tracking producing anterior knee pain (Mohiuddin et al. 2014; Ahmed et al. 2019).

On the increased incidence of knee osteoarthritis reported in association with Müller-Weiss disease, Maceira and Rochera believed it to be secondary to impaired mechanics of the whole limb rather than a primary knee dysplasia. Purportedly, subtalar varus removes shock absorption at the subtalar joint during heel strike and midfoot compensation in the sagittal plane, thereby forcing the extensor mechanism of the knee to compensate for subtalar rigidity with every step. Many of their patients had already undergone total knee replacement prior to presentation with foot problems (Monteagudo and Maceira 2019).

Based on their theory of nutritional deficiency as a major contributing factor, Maceira and Rochera advise ruling out any environmental, socio-economic factors or other systemic disease. Look also for dental caries and enamel hypoplasia with eventual severe loss of dentition by the third decade of life.

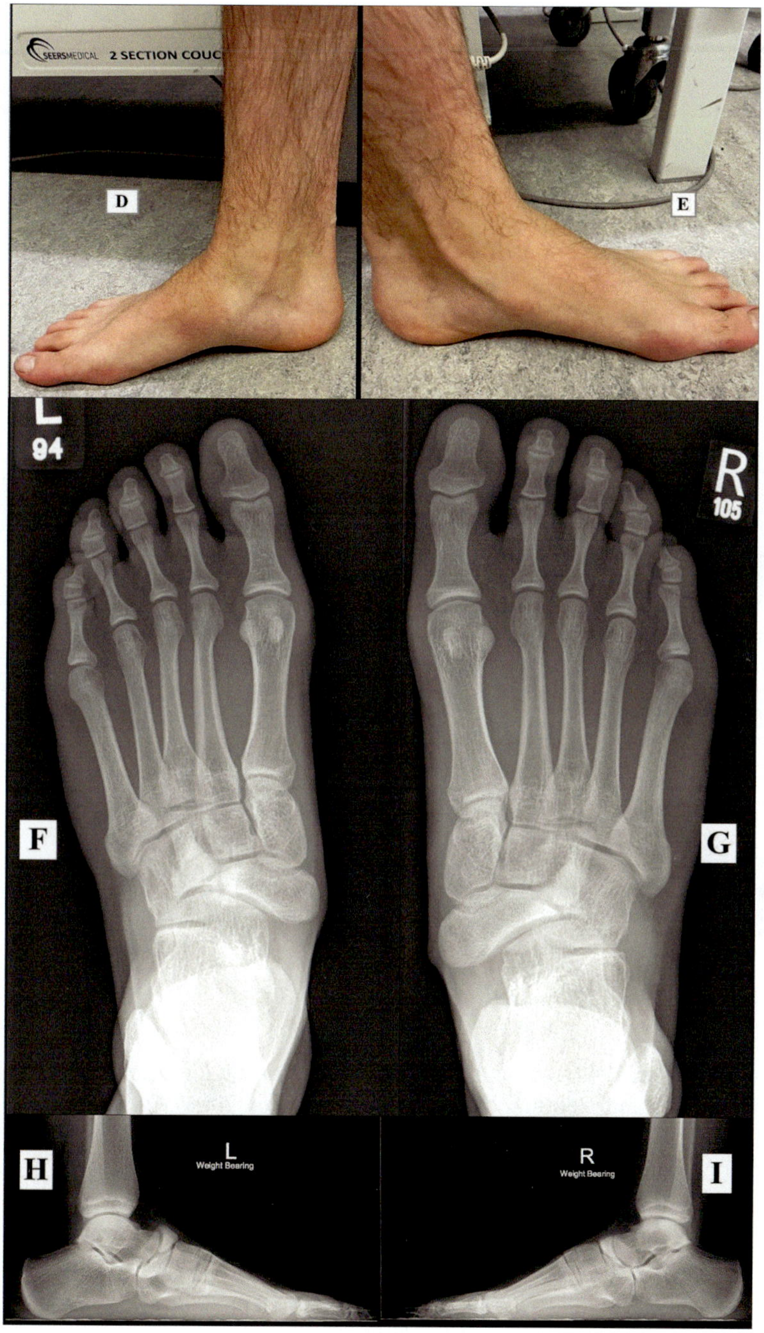


**Fig. 2.2** (continued)

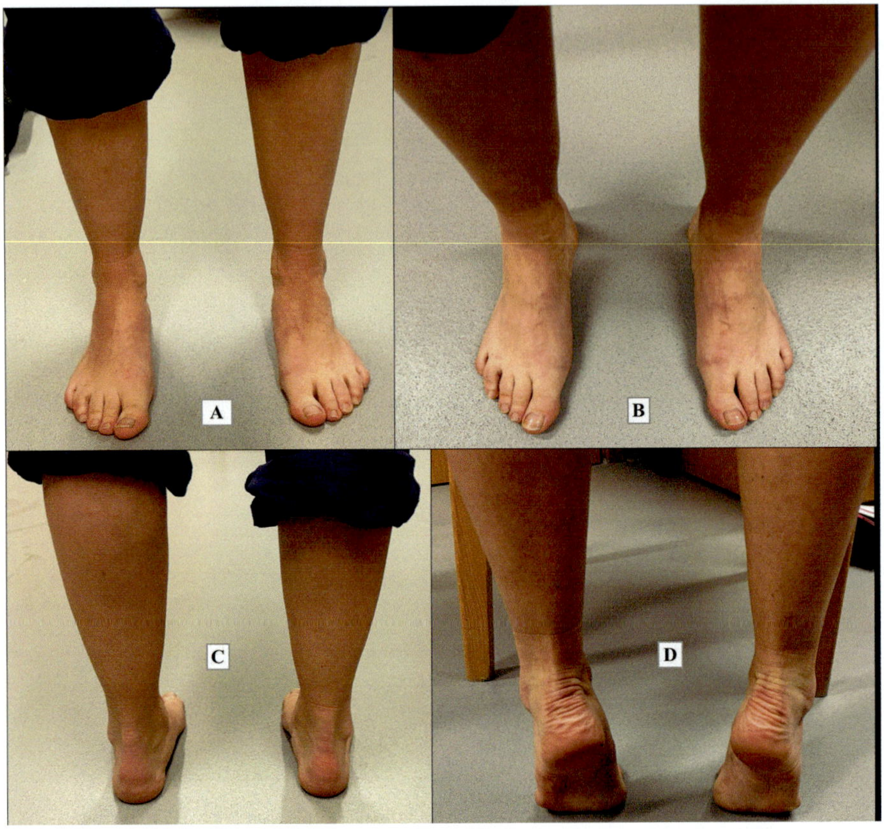


**Fig. 2.3** Asymptomatic feet in a 36-year-old woman. (A) Viewed at ankle level, peekaboo sign is negative. (B) False positive heel varus when viewed from above. (C) Rear view reveals bilateral physiological heel valgus. (D) Both heels normally varize and arches rise when standing on tiptoes

## 2.5 Differential Diagnosis

(a) Köhler's disease is a spontaneous osteochondrosis with different epidemiological, clinical and radiographic features (Sharp et al. 2003). Unilateral in 75–80% of cases, it affects children aged 3–7 years old and occurs mostly in boys with a preponderance of 4:1–6:1. On the other hand, Müller-Weiss disease is frequently bilateral and occurs more often in women with a female to male ratio of 6:4. The navicular appears hypoplastic and flattened on plain radiographs with irregular central sclerosis. It is a benign and self-limiting condition with full clinical and radiological recovery of the navicular. Not uncommonly asymptomatic, it produces only minor symptoms whereas Müller-Weiss disease can cause severe symptoms, disability and progressive deformity.

(b) Stress fractures of the navicular in athletes are typically incomplete and affect the dorsal aspect of the bone (see Chap. 13 on Future Directions).
(c) Concentric osteoarthritis of the talonavicular joint rules out the diagnosis of Müller-Weiss disease, which exhibits an eccentric pattern of degeneration.
(d) Charcot neuropathy.
(e) Osteomyelitis.
(f) Paget's disease.
(g) Osteonecrosis secondary to renal failure.
(h) Inflammatory disease such as rheumatoid arthritis and systemic lupus erythrematosus.
(i) Osteochondritis dissecans affects the talar side of the navicular and does not cause deformity.
(j) Other causes of flatfoot.

**Concluding Remarks**

The catchy term 'pes paradoxical pes planus varus' has perpetuated the myth of mandatory heel varus in Müller-Weiss disease. It appears to have been based (a) on eliciting the peekaboo sign from an elevated viewing point, (b) palpation of the heel when standing on tiptoes and (c) on the assumption that, since the heel moves into valgus as the talar head points medially in progressive collapsing foot deformity, it follows that the heel must automatically move into varus as part of the acetabulum pedis when the talar head shifts laterally as in Müller-Weiss disease.

With the patient standing with both feet at shoulder width, the medial border of both feet parallel and the toes pointing straight ahead at the examiner, the peekaboo sign should be elicited by viewing down the corridor so formed at ankle level, and not at knee level. Palpation for heel varus is best performed with the patient sitting or supine, holding the heel in the examiner's cupped hand, the ankle held in dorsiflexion, gently moving the hindfoot into eversion and assessing spatial orientation of the heel.

Correct assessment of heel position is relevant especially when considering embarking on lateral displacement calcaneal osteotomy as sole surgical treatment for Müller-Weiss disease. If in doubt, hindfoot alignment radiographs will confirm exact heel position.

## References

Ahmed AA, Kandil MI, Tabl EA, Elgazzar AS. Müller-Weiss disease: a topical review. Foot Ankle Int. 2019;40(12):1447–57. https://doi.org/10.1177/1071100719877000.

Ahmed AA, Kandil MI, Tabl EA. Preliminary outcomes of calcaneal lengthening in adolescent flatfoot in Müller-Weiss disease. Foot Ankle Int. 2019;40(7):803–7. https://doi.org/10.1177/1071100719833928

Angthong C, Younger ASE, Chuckpaiwong B, Harnroongroj T, Veljkovic A. A novel update on the management of Müller-Weiss disease: Presentation of a treatment algorithm. Cartilage. 2023:19476035231205684. https://doi.org/10.1177/19476035231205684. Epub ahead of print.

Bartolotta RJ, McCullion JC, Belfi LM, Hentel KD. Mueller-Weiss syndrome: imaging and implications. Clin Imaging. 2014;38(6):895–8. https://doi.org/10.1016/j.clinimag.2014.06.012.
Brailsford JF. Osteochondritis of the adult tarsal navicular. J Bone Joint Surg. 1939;21(1):111–20.
Chiavegatti R, Canales P, Saldias E, Isidro A. Earliest probable case of Mueller-Weiss disease from ancient Egypt. J Foot Ankle Surg. 2018;57(5):1034–6. https://doi.org/10.1053/j.jfas.2018.03.004.
De Fine LE. On bipartite os naviculare pedis. Acta Radiol. 1941;22:377–82.
Doyle T, Napier RJ, Wong-Chung J. Recognition and management of Müller-Weiss disease. Foot Ankle Int. 2012;33(4):275–81. https://doi.org/10.3113/FAI.2012.0275.
Eloundou P, Azankpan E, Bebey F. Le syndrome de Muller-Weiss chez un sujet amateur de tennis. RAFMI. 2020;7(2–1):87–9.
Fornaciari P, Gilgen A, Zwicky L, Horn Lang T, Hintermann B. Isolated talonavicular fusion with tension band for Müller-Weiss syndrome. Foot Ankle Int. 2014;35(12):1316–22. https://doi.org/10.1177/1071100714548197.
Frigg A, Nigg B, Davis E, Pederson B, Valderrabano V. Does alignment in the hindfoot radiograph influence dynamic foot-floor pressures in ankle and tibiotalocalcaneal fusion? Clin Orthop Relat Res. 2010;468(12):3362–70. https://doi.org/10.1007/s11999-010-1449-7
Hetsroni I, Nyska M, Ayalon M. Plantar pressure distribution in patients with Müller-Weiss disease. Foot Ankle Int. 2007;28(2):237–41. https://doi.org/10.3113/FAI.2007.0237.
Maceira E, Rochera R. Müller-Weiss disease: clinical and biomechanical features. Foot Ankle Clin. 2004;9(1):105–25. https://doi.org/10.1016/S1083-7515(03)00153-0.
Manoli AII, Graham B. The subtle cavus foot, "the underpronator", a review. Foot Ankle Int. 2005;26(3):256–63.
Manoli AII, Smith DG, Hansen ST Jr. Scarred muscle excision for the treatment of established ischemic contracture of the lower extremity. Clin Orthop. 1993;292:309–14.
Mohiuddin T, Jennison T, Damany D. Müller-Weiss disease—review of current knowledge. Foot Ankle Surg. 2014;20(2):79–84. https://doi.org/10.1016/j.fas.2013.11.001.
Monteagudo M, Maceira. Management of Müller-Weiss disease. Foot Ankle Clin. 2019;24(1):89–105. https://doi.org/10.1016/j.fcl.2018.09.006
Mueller-Weiss disease. NORD. September 2022. http://www.rarediseases.org
Roy N. What is Mueller-Weiss syndrome, the foot injury Rafael Nadal suffers from? 2022-06-5. http://www.sporskeeda.com
Sharp RJ, Calder JD, Saxby TS. Osteochondritis of the navicular: a case report. Foot Ankle Int. 2003;24(6):509–13. https://doi.org/10.1177/107110070302400611.
Wong-Chung J, Walls A, Lynch-Wong M, Cassidy R, McKenna R, Wilson A, Stephens M. Towards understanding Müller-Weiss disease from an analysis of 95 cases. Foot Ankle Surg. 2023;29(5):401–11. https://doi.org/10.1016/j.fas.2023.05.004.
Yuan C, Wang C, Zhang C, Huang J, Wang X, Ma X. Derotation of the talus and arthrodesis treatment of stages II-V Müller-Weiss disease: midterm results of 36 cases. Foot Ankle Int. 2019;40(5):506–14. https://doi.org/10.1177/1071100719829457.
Zhang MZ, Yu GR. Surgical treatment for Müller-Weiss disease. Foot Ankle Orthop. 2017;2(3). https://doi.org/10.1177/2473011417S000430
Zhang MZ, Yu GR. Surgical treatment for Müller-Weiss disease. Foot Ankle Orthop. 2018;3(3). https://doi.org/10.1177/2473011418S00536

# Chapter 3
# Radiographic Features

**Abstract** The diagnosis of Müller-Weiss disease rests on the finding of compression of the lateral part of the navicular giving it a comma-shaped or hour-glass appearance on weight-bearing plain radiographs. Its medial pole subluxes and extrudes medially while the talar head shifts laterally with resultant decrease in Kite's angle. The second metatarsal is commonly longer than the first. Other radiographic signs are broken cyma lines, striking parallelism of the metatarsals, hallucal sesamoids sitting in "too pretty" position, cuboid sign indicating medial subluxation at the calcaneocuboid joint, an open sinus tarsi indicative of subtalar inversion and varying degrees of midfoot abduction. Méary's angle forms the basis for Maceira's classification, its end-stage V marked by formation of the talocuneiform articulation. Of the adjunctive imaging modalities, SPECT-CT is preferable to MRI for studying arthritis of the various perinavicular joints and remaining bone stock. The hindfoot alignment radiograph is useful for verifying heel position. One study found heel varus in only 33%, heel varus together with flatfoot in 26%, the commonest combination being of heel valgus and flatfoot at 56%. Weight-bearing CT may prove useful in understanding why not all heels move into varus within the acetabulum pedis, when the talar head shifts laterally.

**Keywords** Müller-Weiss disease · Comma-shaped navicular · Cyma lines · Talocuneiform articulation · Méary's angle · Heel varus

## Introduction

According to Arandes and Viladot, "clinical findings are nothing, radiology is everything" in Köhler's disease (Arandes and Viladot 1956). In Müller-Weiss disease, Maceira and Rochera remarked that "clinical findings may be helpful but plain weight-bearing radiographs of the feet are the basic tools for diagnosis (Maceira and Rochera 2004)."

This Chapter details the findings on plain radiographs, which provide the key to diagnosis and clues to pathomechanics of the disease. The role of special

© The Author(s), under exclusive license to Springer Nature Switzerland AG 2024 
J. Wong-Chung, *Comprehensive Guide to Müller-Weiss Disease*,
https://doi.org/10.1007/978-3-031-66644-5_3

investigations in management and future research into the condition are also discussed.

## 3.1 Radiographic Views

Standard hindfoot and forefoot radiographic series include anteroposterior standing radiographs of both ankles, hindfoot alignment views, lateral standing radiographs of both ankles and feet, dorsoplantar standing and medial oblique views of both feet.

Always image the contralateral foot for comparison and to rule out pathology. To avoid parallax error, each foot is imaged separately. For the hindfoot alignment view, the patient stands with the foot placed in neutral position using the medial ± lateral calcaneal contour as guide. The toes point straight ahead. The tube is aimed forward 20° towards the floor and aligned with the tibia and second ray. The image should capture the calcaneum and at least half of the tibia for accuracy.

## 3.2 Radiographic Findings

Many of the radiographic features described below indicate subtalar inversion (Maceira and Rochera 2004; Welck et al. 2016; Wong-Chung et al. 2021).

### *3.2.1 Findings on Dorsoplantar Weight-Bearing Radiographs*

**Hindfoot**

- Reduced Kite's angle or decreased talocalcaneal divergence. The talar head points laterally instead of medially and overlies the anterior calcaneal process instead of beside it (Fig. 3.1).
- Short "S" cyma line with an abrupt inflection at its mid portion, since the talar head no longer lies next to the anterior process of the calcaneus. In a well-aligned foot, the cyma line normally appears as a smooth and unbroken italic S-shaped line formed by the curved joint lines of the talonavicular and calcaneocuboid articulations (Fig. 3.1).
- Apparent widening of talar head due to degenerative changes and altered rotation in the coronal plane.

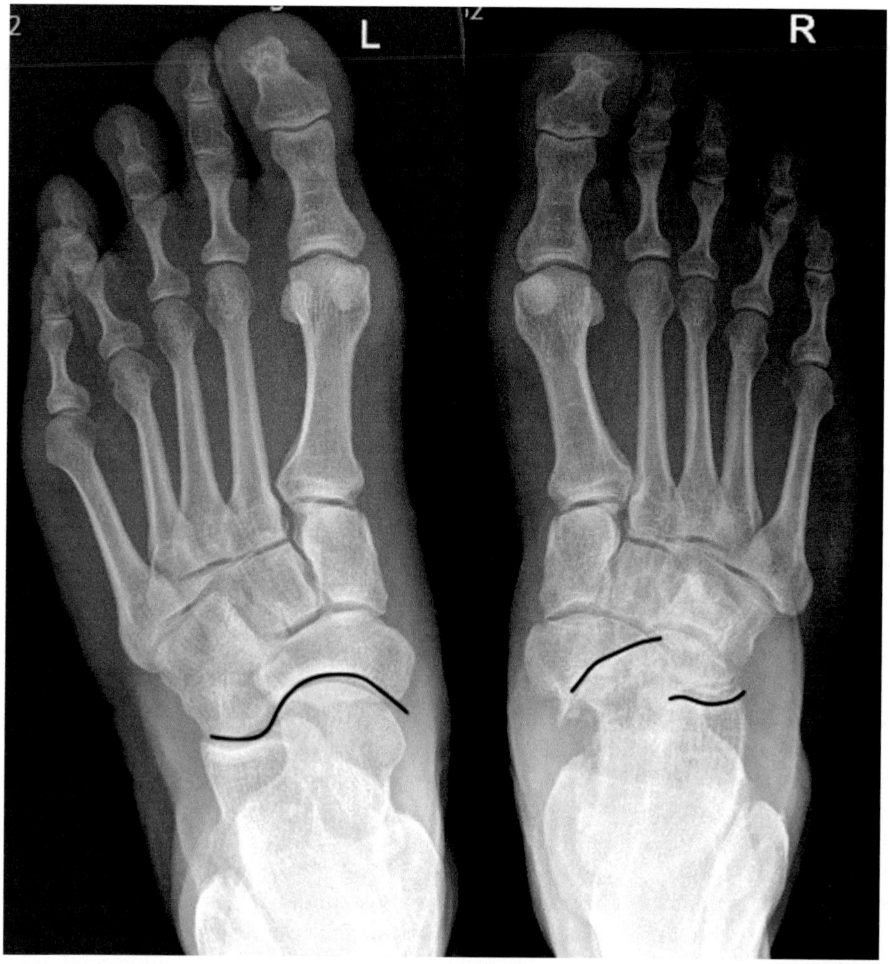


**Fig. 3.1** Dorsoplantar standing radiographs of both feet of a 55-year-old man with Group 3B Maceira Stage V Müller-Weiss disease of the right foot. Compression and fragmentation of the lateral navicular with formation of a talocuneiform articulation. 'Comma-shaped' navicular. Advanced arthritis at the talonavicular joint. Medial talonavicular subluxation, medial extrusion of the medial navicular pole and medial column shortening. Note the broken 'cyma' line on the right compared to a smooth S-shaped 'cyma' line on the normal left side. The right talar head points laterally instead of medially. It overlies the anterior calcaneal process instead of beside it as on the normal left side. Decreased right Kite's talocalcaneal angle with the longitudinal axis of the talus parallel to that of the calcaneum. Apparent widening of the right talar head. Parallelism of the metatarsals. Diarthrodial joint between the bases of the right first and second metatarsals. 'Elephant's foot' appearance of the base of the first metatarsal. Sesamoids sitting in 'too pretty' position

## Midfoot

- Compression (decreased anteroposterior dimension) of the navicular at the level of the lateral naviculocuneiform joint (NC3) more than at NC2, producing the characteristic 'comma-shaped' or 'hourglass-shaped' navicular (Fig. 3.2A).
- Medial talonavicular subluxation or internal rotation of the medial navicular causing apparent medial extrusion of the navicular tuberosity (Wong-Chung et al. 2021) with resultant medial column shortening.
- Midfoot abduction as measured by the dorsoplantar talo-first metatarsal angle.
- Fracture occurred in half of Maceira's cases (Maceira and Rochera 2004) and 38% of Wong-Chung et al. (2021). It occurs either at the level of the third or second cuneiform bone or the lateral intercuneiform joint. The smaller lateral bone fragment may be clearly seen at times and at other times appear as a subtle shadow that is difficult to distinguish from the underlying cuboid.
- Increased density of the lateral navicular, although this may be apparent rather than real due to superimposition of the navicular and talar head.
- Difficulty in distinguishing the lateral navicular from the underlying cuboid.
- Cuboid sign: medial subluxation of the cuboid (Figs. 3.2A, 3.3A).
- Contour of the Chopart joint line resembles a 'question mark' instead of the typical small 'v'.
- Contact between the talar head and lateral cuneiforms in Maceira Stage V disease—the talocuneiform articulation (Fig. 3.3A-B).
- Arthritis in the perinavicular joints, namely the talonavicular ± naviculocuneiform joints.

## Forefoot

- Short first metatarsal. This may be real or apparent due to internal rotation of the navicular with relative shortening of whole medial column.
- Striking parallelism of the metatarsals, particularly of the first and second, with reduced divergence between first and fifth.
- Cortical hypertrophy of second metatarsal from increased load transmission.
- Variable atrophy of the fourth, and sometimes of the first, third and fifth metatarsals can be particularly noticeable especially when the second is hypertrophied.
- First tarsometatarsal (TMT1) joint lies in a plane perpendicular to the axis of the foot instead of facing medially (Fig. 3.1).
- TMT2 and TMT3 are externally rotated instead of lying perpendicular to axis of the foot.
- Presence of a diarthrodial joint between the bases of the first and second metatarsals. The wide base of the first metatarsal and the perpendicular disposition of its proximal articular surface has been likened to an 'elephant's foot' (Fig. 3.1) by Maceira and Rochera (Maceira and Rochera 2004).
- Sesamoids tend to sit in a "too pretty" position beneath the first metatarsal head (Maceira and Rochera 2004).

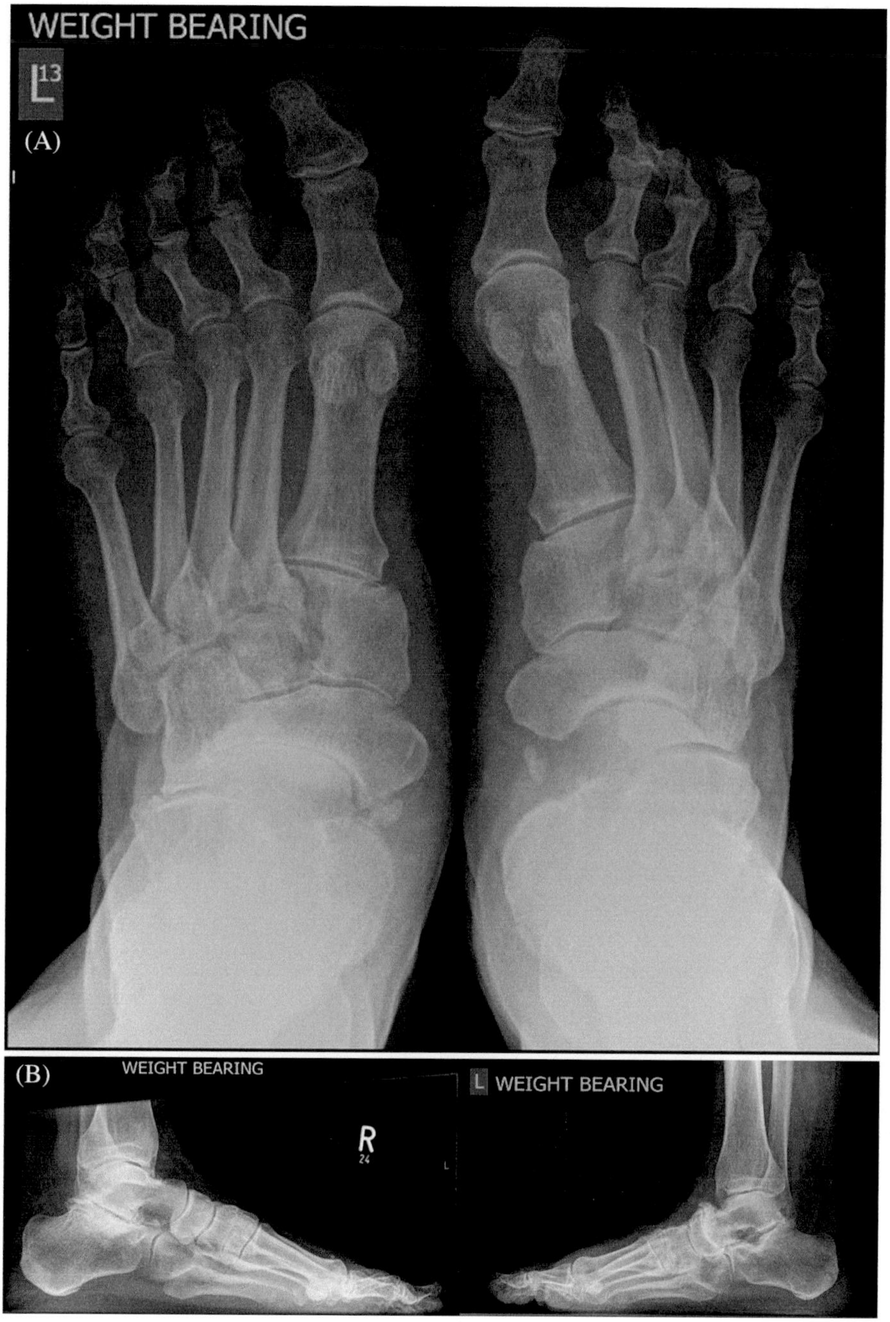
WEIGHT BEARING
L13
(A)
(B)
WEIGHT BEARING
R
L WEIGHT BEARING

◀**Fig. 3.2** (A) Dorsoplantar standing radiographs of both feet of a 48-year-old man with left Group 3B Maceira Stage III disease affecting the talonavicular more than the naviculocuneiform joints. Cuboid sign. Hypertrophied second metatarsal is longer than the first. (B) Lateral standing radiographs demonstrating a sinus tarsi "see-through" sign, decreased calcaneal pitch, decreased talocalcaneal divergence, retropositioning of the fibula and advanced osteoarthritis at the talonavicular joint with dorsal osteophyte formation. Méary's angle is neutral. In this case, cyma lines appear symmetrical on both affected and unaffected sides. (C) Axial CT slice reveals advanced talonavicular arthritis with formation of subchondral cysts communicating with the middle naviculocuneiform (NC) joint. Pain and tenderness were also present at the naviculocuneiform joints. (D) T1-weighted MRI coronal images demonstrating altered signal changes at NC2 and NC3

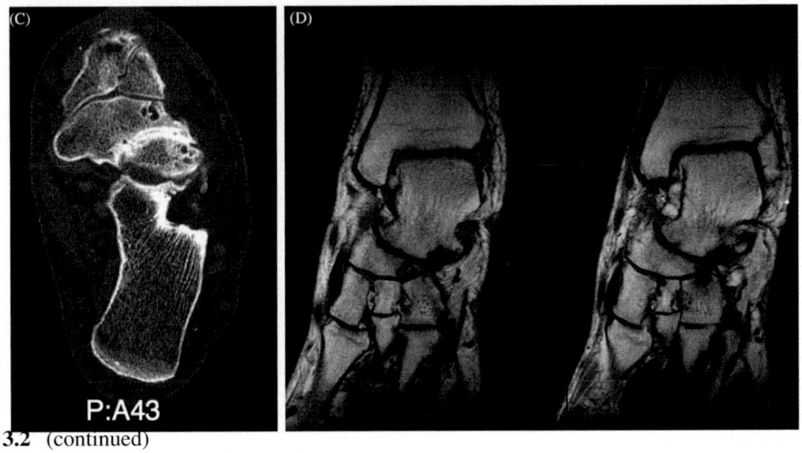


**Fig. 3.2** (continued)

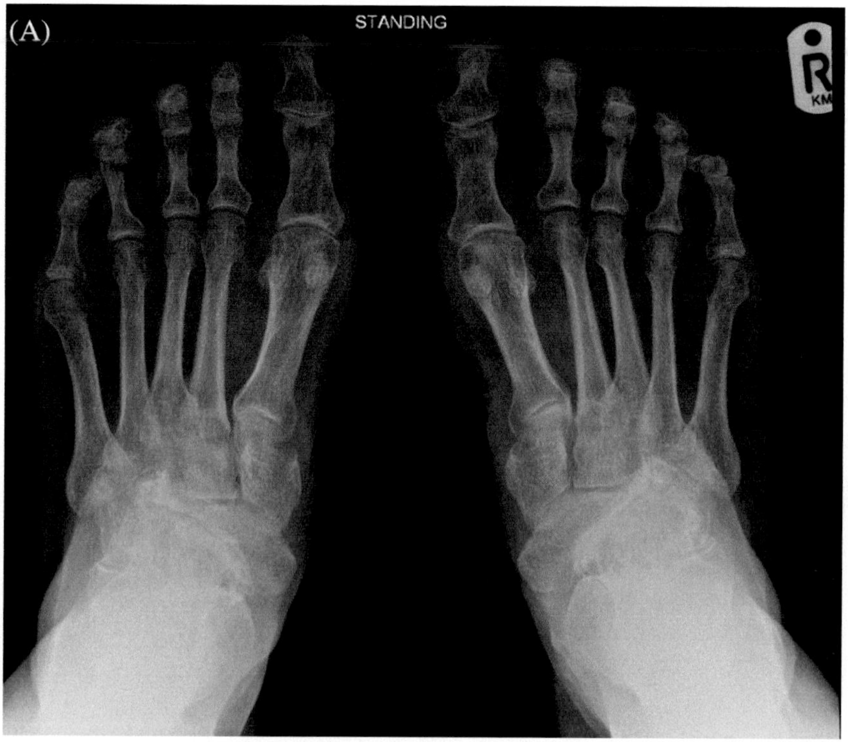


**Fig. 3.3** (A) Dorsoplantar standing radiographs of a 62-year-old male farmer with bilateral Group 3B Maceira Stage V Müller-Weiss disease. Compression and fragmentation of the lateral navicular with medial talonavicular subluxation. Bilateral 'cuboid' signs. Second metatarsal is longer than the first. (B) Talocuneiform articulations on medial oblique views. (C) Dorsal extrusion of the lateral navicular fragments with sagging at the talonavicular joints, more marked on the left. Broken 'cyma' lines. Harris lines in both distal tibiae. Note also prominent inferior border of cuboid bones bilaterally as referred to in Sect. 2.3.2. (D) Hindfoot alignment radiographs show valgus offset of the left heel and neutral position of the right heel. (E) SPECT-CT shows advanced degeneration with marked radioisotope uptake at both talonavicular joints. Fragmentation of the lateral navicular with irregularity of its distal surface at the lateral more than at the middle naviculocuneiform joints. (F) Long axial WBCT slice confirms reveals advanced degeneration at both talonavicular joints, compression and fragmentation of the lateral navicular, medial extrusion of their medial poles and established degeneration at the resulting left talocuneiform articulation. Weight-bearing CT (WBCT) with 3D reconstructions. Dorsal view through (G) X-Ray sharp (H) Bones and (I) Skin windows. (J) Frontal view using skin window. The feet are not pointing straight ahead. Rear view through all windows, (K) X-Ray sharp (L) Bones and (M) Skin, confirm valgus offset of the left heel and a neutral right heel

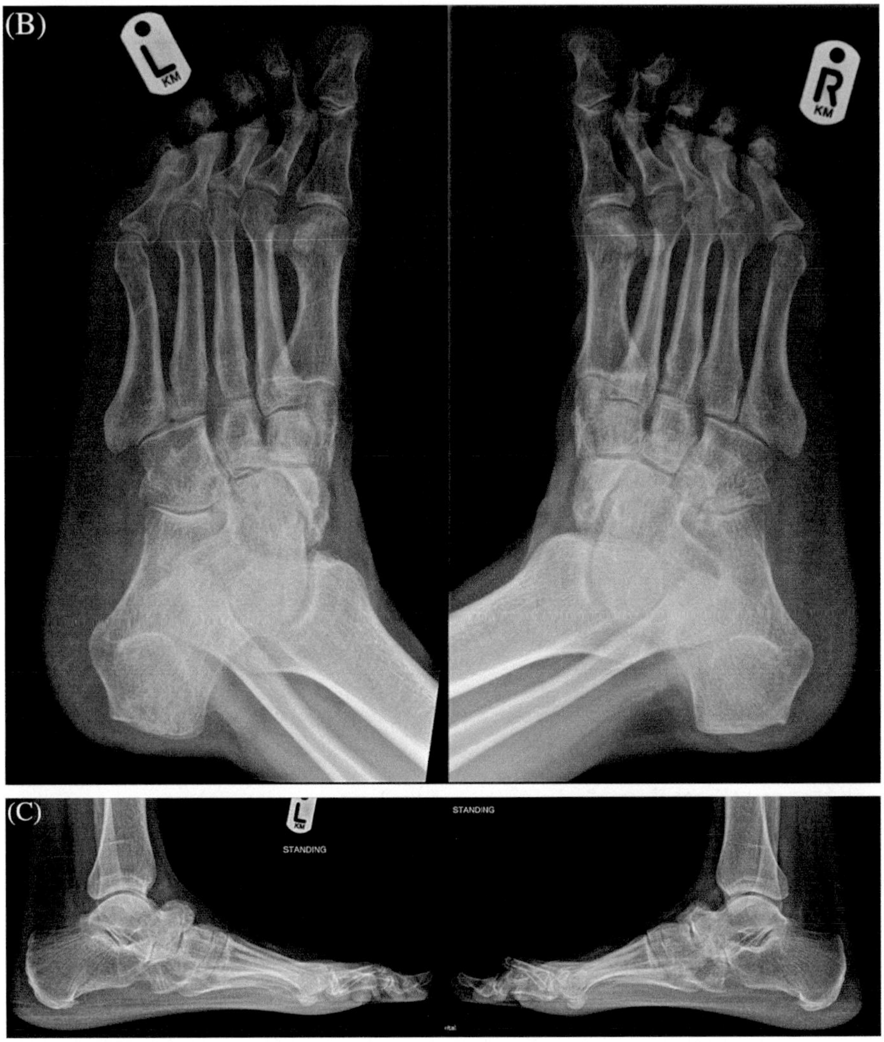


**Fig. 3.3** (continued)

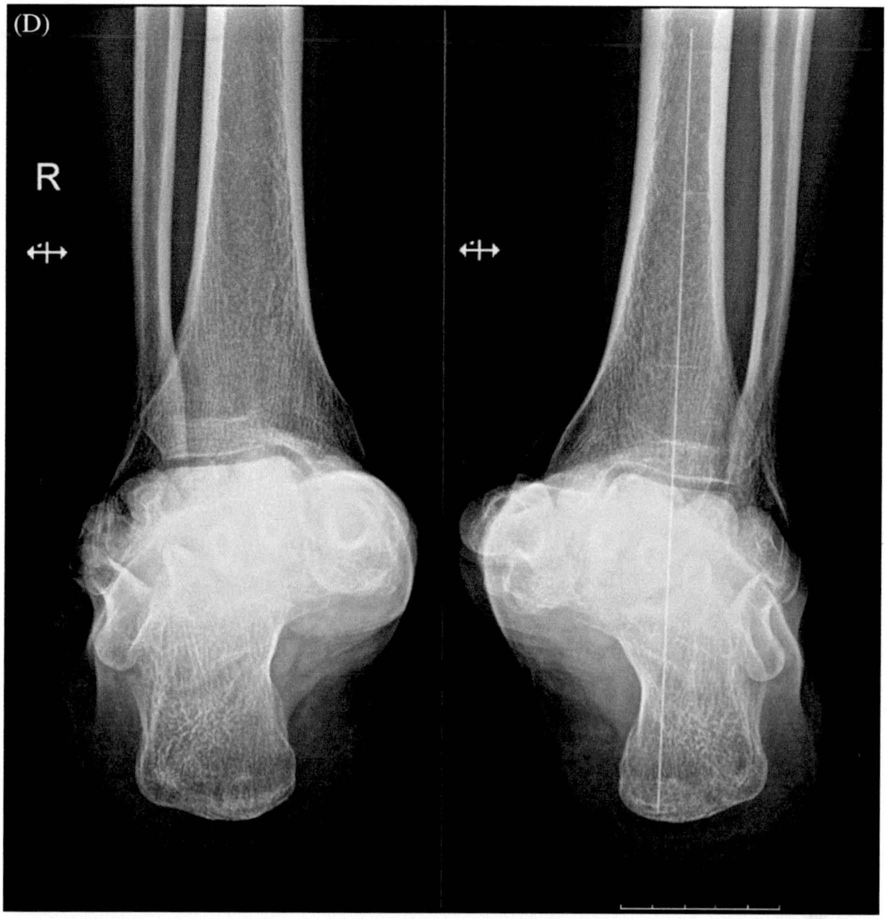


**Fig. 3.3** (continued)

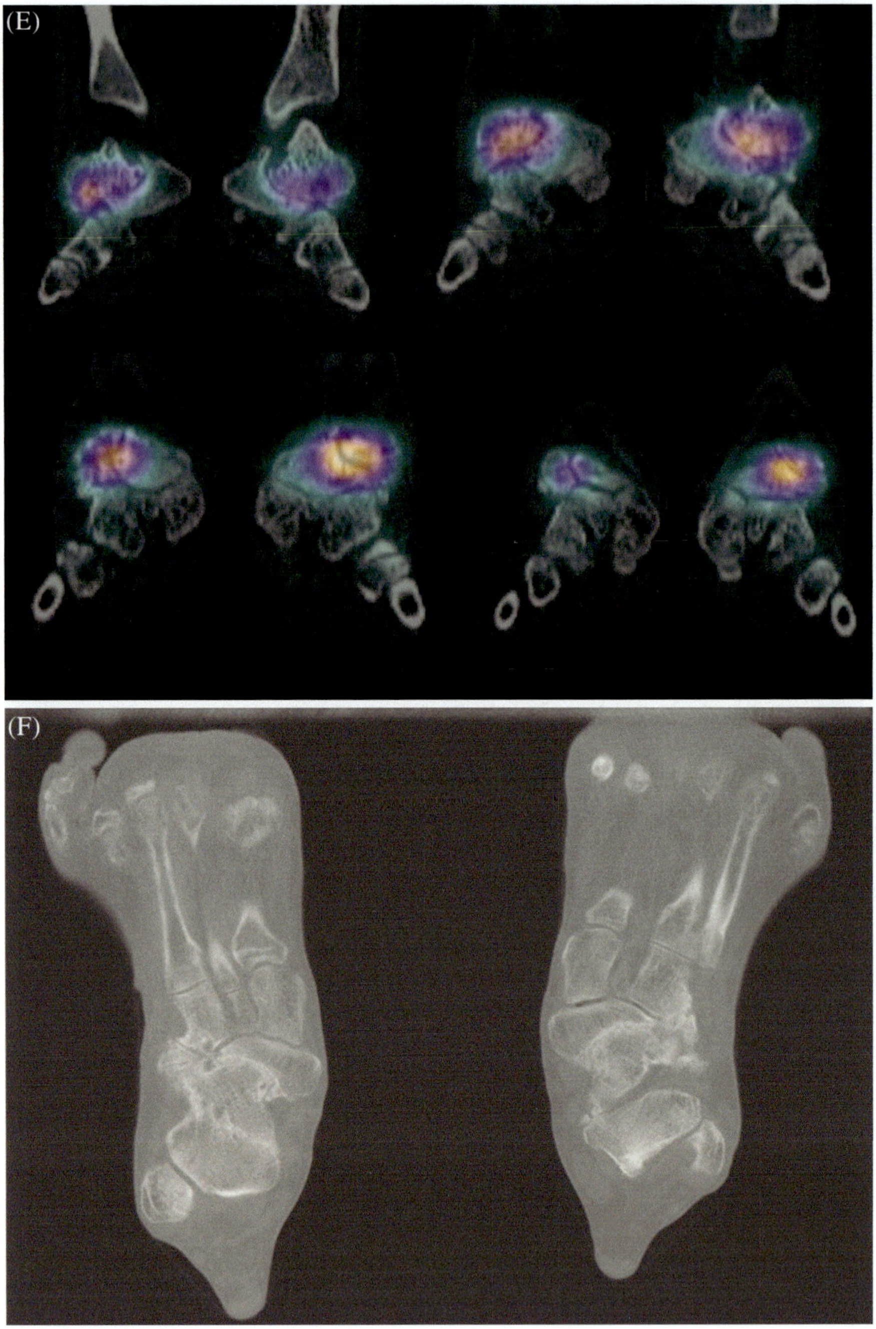


**Fig. 3.3** (continued)

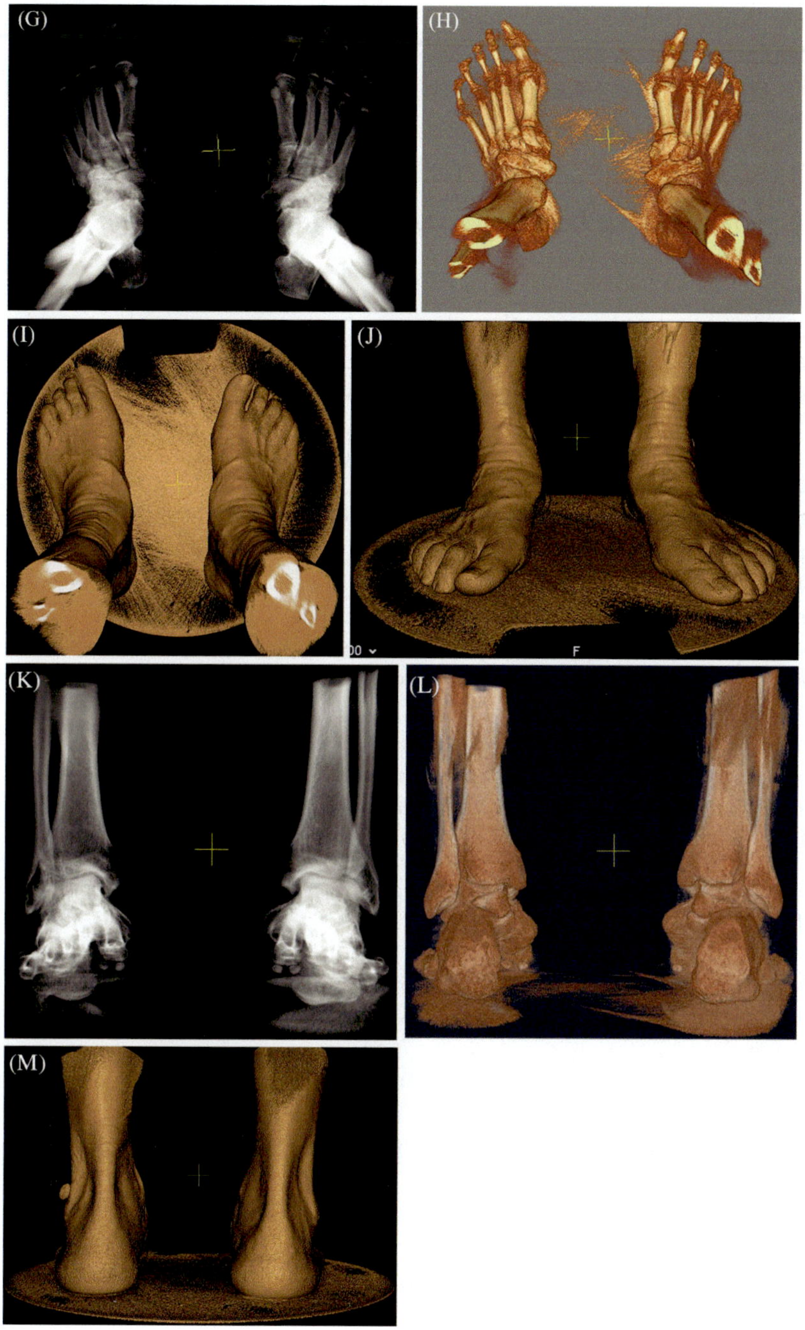


**Fig. 3.3** (continued)

- Low incidence of hallux valgus. A few of Maceira's patients complained of prominent bunions. Increased distal metatarsal articular angle in these feet was instrumental in causing overcorrection following first ray surgery with poor outcomes.

### 3.2.2 *Findings on Lateral Weight-Bearing Radiographs*

**Hindfoot**

- Sinus tarsi "see-through" sign represents an enlarged sinus tarsi secondary to hindfoot varus placing its longitudinal axis in the same plane as the X-ray beam (Fig. 3.2B).
- Posterior and middle subtalar facets visible on the same view.
- Decreased calcaneal pitch.
- Decreased talocalcaneal divergence angle with the axis of talus and calcaneus tending to run parallel.
- Elongated italic '*S*' cyma line since there is little if any overlapping between the talar head and anterior process of the calcaneum. The talar head lies above and not adjacent to the anterior calcaneal process.
- Double shadow of talar dome and retropositioning of the fibula due to external rotation of the hindfoot (Fig. 3.2B).
- Soft tissue shadow at the back of the heel may appear to protrude posteriorly due to apparent anterior advancement of the ankle relative to the foot.
- Prominent anterior border of cuboid (Figs. 3.2B and 3.3C)
- Harris lines may be present (Fig. 3.3C).

**Midfoot**

- Decreased anteroposterior dimension of the navicular.
- Méary's angle to determine Maceira stage (See Chap. 4 on Classification Systems).
- Fragmentation of the navicular with fracture line running from dorsal/distal to plantar/proximal.
- Dorsal extrusion of the dorsolateral fragment of the navicular (Fig. 3.3C).
- Perinavicular osteoarthritis.

### 3.2.3 *Brailsford's Osteochondritis*

It is worth mentioning that Brailsford had already described many of the above-listed radiographic features in 1935, not long after Wilhem Röentgen had first discovered X-rays on November 8, 1895 (Brailsford 1939). The reader is referred to a complete description of Brailsford's contributions in Chap. 1. He termed the condition an osteochondritis, believing the separated lateral navicular fragment resembled the osteochondritis dissecans described earlier by Franz König at the medial femoral condyle.

Here are some of Brailsford's key points:

- Frequently bilateral, it occurred in women only.
- Less extensive changes on one side ranged from 'mere compression of the plastic outer third of the navicular' to compression of the lateral half 'to about two-thirds of the thickness of the normal medial half'.
- On the more severe side, the navicular was split obliquely into 2 parts through its middle third. A sagittal cleft ran from the dorsal distal surface of the navicular to the midpoint of the talonavicular joint.
- Separation of the fragments occurred with 'listhesis' or 'gliding' of the navicular 'in a proximal direction over the medial surface of the talar head'. Brailsford was describing medial talonavicular subluxation, which approached near to complete dislocation in some cases.
- In describing how the axis of the first metatarsal passed medial to the inner surface of the talar neck, Brailsford was effectively describing the dorsoplantar talo-first metatarsal angle, as we know and use it today for assessment of midfoot abduction.
- The medial fragment displaced not only medially, but also inferiorly with collapse of the medial longitudinal arch.
- The lateral fragment drifted laterally and dorsally to overlie the dorsal surface of the lateral and middle cuneiforms.
- Decrease in distance between the talar head and middle/lateral cuneiforms as a result of this 'listhesis' culminating in some instances with direct articulation of the talar head with the lateral and middle cuneiforms—the talocuneiform articulation that characterizes Maceira Stage V Müller-Weiss disease (Maceira and Rochera 2004).
- Short first metatarsal. Hypertrophied second metatarsal. Slender atrophied third, fourth and fifth metatarsals.
- Gradual increase in compression and talonavicular subluxation with resultant increase in separation of the 2 navicular fragments.
- Severe osteoarthritis at the midfoot joints in late stages, including at the calcaneocuboid and first tarsometatarsal articulations in some feet.

### 3.2.4 Bipartite Navicular

Timeline of introduction of the term bipartite navicular closely paralleled that of Brailsford's osteochondritis (Volk 1937). It soon became apparent that both terms were describing the same condition. And some authors even used the terms Brailsford's disease, osteochondritis, bipartite navicular and Müller-Weiss disease interchangeably, implying synonymity of all 4 appellations (Wiley and Brown 1981). This author opines that the severe forms of Brailsford's osteochondritis and bipartite navicular represent Stage V of Maceira's classification of Müller-Weiss disease. This is discussed at length in Chap. 1, Sects. 1.7 and 1.8).

## 3.3 MRI

In the early stage of the disease, MRI detects homogenous loss of bone marrow signal intensity in the dorsolateral part of the navicular on T1-weighted images, effusion in adjacent joints and bone marrow oedema on short tau inversion recovery (STIR) sequences. MRI cannot differentiate between changes due to primary or secondary osteonecrosis.

It has been postulated that excessive mechanical strain may cause increased intraosseous pressure and disrupt the blood supply to the lateral navicular. Welck et al. deemed it unlikely that primary osteonecrosis can cause hindfoot varus and rotation of the talar head. They argued that subtalar varus is already present in Stage I, when there is minimal necrosis. They surmised that osteonecrosis is the result rather than the cause of deformity (Welck et al. 2016).

Instead of MRI (Fig. 3.2D), this author now prefers SPECT-CT for special imaging of Müller-Weiss feet.

## 3.4 SPECT-CT

When established changes are evident on plain radiographs, SPECT-CT offers more useful information and helps in selection of which joints to fuse. Information obtainable from the CT component include morphological changes in the navicular bone, degree of bone destruction, amount of remaining bone stock and bone density, severity of deformity, extent of medial column shortening, degree of degenerative changes in the perinavicular joints, presence and site of fracture or fragmentation, dorsal extrusion of the dorsolateral fragment, and direct articulation of the talar head with the lateral cuneiform indicative of a Maceira Stage V lesion. It also helps with planning of surgery.

The SPECT component informs of the intensity of metabolic activity at the perinavicular joints, namely the talonavicular, subtalar, calcaneocuboid and naviculocuneiform joints. The degree of radioisotope uptake can be graded according to a colour scale (Fig. 3.3E). For example, on a Siemens Symbia Truepoint machine, an image fusion software (Syngo, Siemens) combines a 16 Bit Warm Metal Colour Scale with an 8 Bit Gray Scale for co-registration of bone SPECT scans with CT to provide colour-graded images. White is graded as 4+ indicating intense $Tc^{99m}$-HDP uptake; yellow as 3+ indicating high uptake; purple-pink as 2+ indicating medium uptake, and blue-green as 1+ indicating low uptake (Wong-Chung et al. 2021).

## 3.5 Weight-Bearing CT

Weight-bearing CT (WBCT) offers all the advantages of conventional CT, but in a functional position. It enables detailed three-dimensional appreciation of the hindfoot deformity, degree of midfoot shortening and collapse in a load bearing position. It is useful for planning surgical reconstruction and fixation of complex and dynamic deformities. It allows exact calculation of how much medial column length needs to be restored at surgery and size of calcaneal osteotomy required to correct alignment (Welck et al. 2016). And like a conventional CT, it provides information on amount of remaining navicular bone stock and density, evaluation of fracture lines and sites of perinavicular arthritis (Fig. 3.3F–M).

Li et al. (2022) obtained WBCT in 17 feet of 12 patients with Müller-Weiss disease and compared alignment of the hindfoot and medial arch against 10 feet with flexible progressive collapsing foot deformity (PCFD) and 10 normal feet (Li et al. 2022). The hindfoot moment arm measured −3.44 mm, 15.75 mm and 3.19 mm in the respective groups, negative values denoting heel varus and positive values indicating heel valgus. Foot and ankle offset was −0.72%, 7.42% and 2.63% respectively. Talonavicular joint coverage angles were −7.18, 22.11 and 11.37; middle facet subluxation 14, 45 and 23%; calcaneocuboid joint subluxation −0.19, 0 and −0.04, positive values indicating lateral subluxation and negative values denoting medial subluxation. Arch height indices were 0.46, 0.45 and 0.58. Differences among the 3 groups reached statistical differences for all parameters, except for middle facet subluxation and fifth metatarsal-medial cuneiform height ratios between Müller-Weiss feet and normal controls.

The authors concluded that hindfoot varus is a typical feature of Müller-Weiss disease. As the talar head rotates laterally, the subtalar joint is driven into varus. This occurs through peritalar subluxation with medial subluxation at both the middle facet and calcaneocuboid joints—opposite to the direction of lateral subluxation in PCFD. No significant difference in the medial arch was detected between the Müller-Weiss feet and normal controls. Structural changes in the mid and hindfoot in Müller-Weiss disease hence differ completely from those found in PCFD.

## 3.6 "Paradoxical Pes Planus Varus": Myth or Fact?

One of the myths that compounds much of the unknown about Müller-Weiss disease is the term "paradoxical pes planus varus." Coined by Maceira and Rochera, it perpetuates the concept of heel varus as a prerequisite for the diagnosis of Müller-Weiss disease, to the point of achieving engraved status from its proponents: "If the heel is not in varus, it is not Müller-Weiss disease."

Motion at the 'acetabulum pedis' permits displacements of the talar head, calcaneus and navicular relative to each other—the talocalcaneonavicular articulation. Since subtalar valgus occurred with displacement of the talar head towards the medial side as in PCFD, Maceira and Rochera assumed that any lateralization of the head of the talus implied subtalar varus. They stated: "Any incompetence of the acetabulum pedis at its lateral end will result in rearfoot varus. MWD is the clinical expression of an acetabular protrusion at the lateral portion of the acetabulum pedis." Three-dimensional CT reconstruction images obtained using Surfdriver software (www.surfdriver.com) demonstrated flattening of the posterior and inferior surface of the lateral half of the navicular (Maceira and Rochera 2004). This allows the talar head to protrude laterally and inferiorly, 'thus inducing subtalar varus'. This assumption may be what led them to assume that all Müller-Weiss feet must have hindfoot varus. Somehow though, as also reported by several other authors, lateralization of the talar head does not always translate into obligatory heel varus, whereas medial displacement of the talar head invariably means hindfoot valgus as seen in PCFD.

Firstly, as correctly pointed out by Ahmed et al., the medial longitudinal arch is apex dorsal in Stage II and neutral in Stages I and III of Maceira's classification (Ahmed et al. 2019a, 2019b; Myerson 2019). Only in Stages IV and V does the arch sag. Secondly, many studies have shown that the heel is not always in varus, having been reported in both neutral and valgus positions.

Therefore, Ahmed et al. go so far as to state that the hallmark deformity is not heel varus, but instead the comma-shaped navicular resulting from compression of its lateral portion, regardless of heel position.

In support of Ahmed et al., physicians and radiologists turn to the dorsoplantar radiograph to make a diagnosis of Müller-Weiss disease, and not to the hindfoot alignment view that many do not even obtain.

Figure 3.3 serves to illustrate a case of bilateral Müller-Weiss disease, in which neither heel is in varus as evidenced by hindfoot alignment views and 3D weight-bearing CT reconstructed images. The left heel is offset in valgus and the right heel is in neutral to slight valgus. (See also Sect. 2.3.1 in Chap. 2 on Clinical Features).

The next section summarizes the results of a radiographic analysis of 68 feet conducted in 2021 by the author.

## 3.7 Obligatory Heel Varus: A Prerequisite for Müller-Weiss Disease?

Maceira and Rochera (2004) are to be commended for their seminal work analysing 191 feet with Müller-Weiss disease and the classification reached therefrom. All patients were said to have heel varus. In another more recent study co-authored by Maceira, all of 14 feet also reportedly had heel varus as measured using Saltzman's method, although no illustrative example or values of heel offset are given. All feet underwent isolated lateral displacement calcaneal osteotomy as sole treatment for Müller-Weiss disease with good outcomes (Avila et al. 2016; Li et al. 2016, 2017). The authors hence considered hindfoot varus to be a hallmark and prerequisite for the diagnosis of Müller-Weiss disease.

Wong-Chung et al. set out to test Maceira's hypotheses of (a) universal heel varus and 'paradoxical pes planus varus' as hallmark deformities of Müller-Weiss disease, (b) of greater sagging of the medial longitudinal arch and (c) greater degree of medial extrusion of the medial navicular pole with increasing amounts of compression and fragmentation of the navicular (Wong-Chung et al. 2021). If, as postulated by Maceira, the talar head moves laterally and inferiorly, driving the subtalar joint into varus and squeezing the medial navicular pole more medially, the angle subtended by the longitudinal axis of the talar neck with the lateral surface of the calcaneum on dorsoplantar radiographs should theoretically decrease with increasing amount of compression and medial extrusion of the navicular. Following on, heel position should shift towards varus offset and the medial arch should sag. Therefore, they also checked for correlations between Kite's AP talocalcaneal angle and (i) degree of compression of the lateral navicular (ii) medial extrusion of the navicular (iii) heel offset and (iv) Méary's angle.

Their study comprised 68 consecutive feet in 19 men and 29 women, aged 14 to 87 (mean, 61 $\pm$ 24) years old. The condition was bilateral in 20, left-sided in 19 and right-sided in 9 patients. Méary's talo-first metatarsal angles were measured on lateral standing radiographs of ankles and feet. Heel offset was measured on the hindfoot alignment view using the method of Saltzman and El-Khoury (Saltzman and El-Khoury 1995).

On dorsoplantar standing radiographs of the feet, the anteroposterior (AP) thickness of the navicular was measured at the thickest part of its medial pole and at the midpoint of each naviculocuneiform (NC) joint along a line perpendicular to the transverse axis of the bone at that point. Percentage compression of the navicular at the level of each NC joint, for example at NC2, then equals $\{\frac{\text{AP thickness at medial pole} - \text{AP thickness at NC2}}{\text{AP thickness at medial pole}} \text{x } 100\}$.

Extrusion of the medial pole of the navicular was defined as the perpendicular distance from the most medial point on the navicular tuberosity to a line joining the medial borders of the talar head and medial cuneiform. Kite's AP talocalcaneal angle was measured on dorsoplantar radiographs as the angle formed between the longitudinal axis of the talus and lateral border of the calcaneum.

The authors found valgus heel offset to be more prevalent than varus heel offset ($p < 0.001$). The heel was in varus in just 33% (range, 1–26 mm; mean, 9 $\pm$ 7.5), in neutral in 2% and in valgus in 65% (range, $-2$ to $-17$ mm; mean, $-8 \pm 4.4$). Only 26% had a combination of heel varus and medial arch sag, the so-called 'paradoxical pes planus varus'. Instead, the commonest combination was of heel valgus and medial arch sag at 56%. These findings do not hence support the term 'paradoxical pes planus varus', coined by Maceira and Rochera as a hallmark characteristic of Müller-Weiss disease.

The medial longitudinal arch sagged in the majority of cases (83%) and was raised in only 9%. Level of sag was at the naviculocuneiform joint in 50 feet (91%) and at the talonavicular joint in 5 feet (9%). Apex of the raised medial arch was at the level of the naviculocuneiform joint in 5 feet and at the talonavicular in 1 foot.

Inverse relationships existed between Méary's angle and the degree of navicular compression reaching statistical significance at NC2 ($r = -0.274$, $p = 0.027$) but not at NC3.

Taking all cases into account, moderate correlation existed between degree of medial extrusion and percentage compression at NC2 ($r = 0.572$, $p < 0.001$) and NC3 ($r = 0.572$, $p < 0.001$). In unilateral cases, the difference in extrusion between the affected and uninvolved sides also showed a strong correlation with the degree of compression at NC2 ($r = 0.637$, $p = 0.001$) and moderate but still significant correlation with degree of compression at NC3 ($r = 0.429$, $p = 0.036$).

In all unilateral cases, extrusion on the affected side was significantly greater than on the contralateral unaffected side ($10.2 \pm 3.4$ mm v/s $6.3 \pm 2.5$ mm; $p = 0.001$). In 15 of the 20 bilateral cases, extrusion was significantly greater on the side with more compression than on the opposite side with less compression ($11 \pm 3.5$ mm v/s $7.9 \pm 2.6$ mm; $p = 0.001$). In the other 5, extrusion was less on the more compressed side than on the opposite side with less compression ($11.3 \pm 2.6$ mm v/s $13.9 \pm 3.2$ mm; $p = 0.006$).

No correlation existed either between Méary's angle and degree of medial extrusion or between Méary's angle and heel alignment.

Significant inverse relationships existed between Kite's angle and percentage compression at both NC2 and NC3 in unilateral and bilateral cases. Similarly, significant inverse relationships occurred between Kite's angle and degree of medial extrusion of the navicular. In 96% of unilateral cases, Kite's angle was significantly lower on the affected side with more extrusion than on the contralateral normal side ($11.1^{\circ} \pm 8.1^{\circ}$ v/s $22.2^{\circ} \pm 7.3^{\circ}$; $p < 0.001$). In 10 of the 20 bilateral cases, Kite's angle is significantly lower on the more extruded side than on the side with less extrusion ($8.8^{\circ} \pm 5.6^{\circ}$ v/s $17.3^{\circ} \pm 9.0^{\circ}$; $p = 0.019$). In the other 10 bilateral cases, Kite's angle was equal or higher on the side with more extrusion than on the opposite side with less extrusion ($14.5^{\circ} \pm 8.7^{\circ}$ v/s $13.1 \pm 8.0^{\circ}$; $p < 0.001$). No correlation was detected between Kite's angle and either heel offset or Méary's angle.

Only 4 feet fitted into Maceira Stage II with heel varus and a positive Méary's angle. Compression averaged 28% at the level of NC2 and 57% at the level of NC3 with associated fracture through the lateral navicular in just 1 of the 4 feet.

Only 1 case corresponded to a Maceira Stage III with heel varus and Méary's angle of 0°. Compression was 35% at the level of NC2 and 64% at the level of NC3.

Fifteen cases fitted into Stages IV and V of Maceira's classification with heel varus and a negative Méary's angle. Compression averaged 36° at the level of NC2 and 61% at the level of NC3 with associated fractures in 7 feet.

Fracture of the navicular was present in 26 of the 68 feet. In these 26 feet, Méary's angle was negative in 84%, positive in 12% and neutral in 4%. The heel was offset in valgus in 62%, neutral in 5% and varus in 33%. Fracture occurred most commonly at the level of the lateral intercuneiform joint or third cuneiform bone. It was incomplete in 5 feet, undisplaced in 5 and displaced by more than 2 mm in 3 feet. Compression in the feet with incomplete and undisplaced fractures averaged 36% at NC2 and 66% at NC3. In the other 13 feet, the lateral fragment was extruded dorsally with the talar head articulating directly with the lateral cuneiform bone, corresponding to Stage

V of Maceira's classification. In these 13 feet, heel offset averaged $-2.6 \pm 9.0$ mm (range, $-16$ to $+$ 14 mm) and Méary's angle averaged $-11^\circ \pm 8.6^\circ$ (range, $8^\circ \pm$ -22°). Percentage compression averaged 48% at NC2 and 85% at NC3.

In conclusion, the study confirms that greater degrees of compression and incidence of fracture occur moving across Maceira Stages II to V.

It partly supports the assumption of more medial arch sag with greater degrees of navicular compression. Although inverse relationships exist between Méary's angle and degree of compression, these only reach statistical significance at NC2, but not at NC3.

It completely validates Maceira's hypothesis of the navicular being compressed laterally and squeezed medialwards, as degree of extrusion of its medial pole correlates moderately to strongly with percentage compression at NC2 and NC3. Extrusion is significantly greater on the involved side in all unilateral cases, and on the side with more compression in 75% of cases. It should be noted that apparent extrusion is due to the medial subluxation at the talonavicular joint and is not an actual squeezing out of bone material.

The study verifies part of Maceira's hypothesized pathomechanism of Müller-Weiss disease. Kite's angle decreases with increasing degree of compression at both NC2 and NC3 in both unilateral and bilateral cases. Kite's angle also correlates inversely with increasing degree of extrusion. It is significantly lower on the affected side in 96% of unilateral cases and on the side with more extrusion in 50% of bilateral cases. In other words, observed reductions in Kite's talocalcaneal angle confirm that lateral shift and inferior protrusion of the talar head causes increasing compression of the navicular and medial extrusion of its medial pole.

However, lateral shift of the talar head does not always result in heel varus, since there is no correlation between Kite's angle, heel offset and Méary's angle in any combination of 2 variables. This invalidates the other part of the hypothesis that led Maceira and Rochera to coin the term 'paradoxical pes planus varus.' As such, the authors caution against universal advocacy of lateral displacement calcaneal osteotomy, as the heel is not always in varus in Müller-Weiss disease.

Future studies should investigate why the heel is in varus in some cases and valgus in others. Heel position may vary according to age of onset of disease and joints affected.

## Concluding Remarks

Weight-bearing plain radiographs remain the mainstay for initial diagnosis of Müller-Weiss disease. The key diagnostic feature is compression of the lateral part of the navicular giving it a comma-shaped appearance. A common finding is an overlong second metatarsal, which is believed to be responsible for excessive compression of the lateral navicular. The medial pole of the navicular subluxes medially, while the talar head shifts laterally and inferiorly with resultant decrease of Kite's angle and Méary's angle, the latter forming the basis for Maceira's classification.

Of the additional imaging modalities, MRI proves valuable for diagnosis of Maceira Stage I disease, when plain radiographs reveal no bony abnormality. For later stages, it helps to quantify the extent of bone necrosis and degree of degeneration at the perinavicular joints. This Author prefers SPECT-CT to study the amount of bone loss, remaining bone stock and the perinavicular joints.

Hindfoot alignment radiographs are very useful for accurate assessment of heel position. Studies using hindfoot alignment radiographs have demonstrated that the heel is not always in varus in Müller-Weiss disease. Only 33% of cases had heel varus. The combination of heel varus and flatfoot, that would fit the description of a paradoxical pes planus varus, was present in only 26%, the commonest combination being of heel valgus and flatfoot at 56%

Future studies should investigate why the heel does not always move into varus as the talar head shifts laterally, assisted perhaps by weight-bearing CT.

## References

Ahmed AA, Kandil MI, Tabl EA. Preliminary outcomes of calcaneal lengthening in adolescent flatfoot in Müller-Weiss disease. Foot Ankle Int. 2019a;40(7):803–7. https://doi.org/10.1177/1071100719833928.

Ahmed AA, Kandil MI, Tabl EA. Response to "Letter regarding: preliminary outcomes of calcaneal lengthening in adolescent flatfoot in Müller-Weiss disease." Foot Ankle Int. 2019b;40(7):809–10. https://doi.org/10.1177/1071100719849430.

Arandes R, Viladot A. Clínica y tratamiento de las enfermedades del pie. Barcelona:Ed Científico-Médica;1956. p. 257–60.

Avila A, Li S, Myerson M, Maceira E, Monteagudo M. The use of isolated calcaneus osteotomy in the treatment of Müller-Weiss disease. Foot Ankle Surg. 2016;22(2):83. https://doi.org/10.1016/j.fas.2016.05.209.

Brailsford JF. Osteochondritis of the adult tarsal navicular. J Bone Joint Surg. 1939;21(1):111–20.

Li S, Myerson MS, Monteagudo M, Maceira E. The use of calcaneus osteotomy for treatment of symptomatic Muller Weiss disease. Foot Ankle Orthop. 2016;1(1). https://doi.org/10.1177/2473011416S00104

Li S, Myerson MS, Netto CDC. Hindfoot varus deformity: an essential but easily neglected pathological change in Müller-Weiss disease. Foot Ankle Orthop. 2022;7(1):2473011421S00043. https://doi.org/10.1177/2473011421S00043

Li S-Y, Myerson MS, Monteagudo M, Maceira E. Efficacy of calcaneus osteotomy for treatment of symptomatic Müller-Weiss disease. Foot Ankle Int. 2017;38(3):261–9. https://doi.org/10.1177/1071100716677741.

Maceira E, Rochera R. Müller-Weiss disease: clinical and biomechanical features. Foot Ankle Clin. 2004;9(1):105–25. https://doi.org/10.1016/S1083-7515(03)00153-0.

Myerson MS. Letter regarding: Preliminary outcomes of calcaneal lengthening in adolescent flatfoot in Müller-Weiss disease. Foot Ankle Int. 2019;40(7):808. https://doi.org/10.1177/1071100719849425.

Saltzman CL, El-Khoury GY. The hindfoot alignment view. Foot Ankle Int. 1995;16(9):572–6. https://doi.org/10.1177/107110079501600911.

Volk C. Zwei fälle von os naviculare pedis bipartitum. Z Orthop Ihre Grenzgeb. 1937;66:396–403.

Welck MJ, Kaplan J, Myerson MS. Müller-Weiss syndrome: radiological features and the role of weightbearing computed tomography scan. Foot Ankle Spec. 2016;9(3):245–51. https://doi.org/10.1177/1938640016630055.

Wiley JJ, Brown DE. The bipartite tarsal scaphoid. J Bone Joint SUrg. 1981;63B(4):583–6.

Wong-Chung J, McKenna R, Tucker A, Gibson D, Datta P. Radiographic analysis of Müller-Weiss disease. Foot Ankle Surg. 2021;27(5):501–9. https://doi.org/10.1016/j.fas.2020.06.009.

# Chapter 4
# Classification Systems

**Abstract** Maceira's classification depends solely on Méary's angle. Although it describes pathomechanics well, it bears no correlation with severity of symptoms and guides neither treatment nor prognosis. Its stage V, marked by a talocuneiform articulation, constitutes a reliable endpoint. Wong-Chung et al. based their grouping system on age of disease onset, a previous radiologically normal navicular, joints affected, dorsoplantar and lateral talo-first metatarsal angles. None of Wong Group 1 early-onset disease has required surgery yet. It has the greatest compression at the lateral naviculocuneiform (NC) joint, greatest medial extrusion and lowest Kite's angle. All are index minus and have fracture at the lateral navicular, except one. Group 2 Müller-Weissoid feet had previously normal naviculars, on average 6 years earlier. Only talonavicular (TN) joint is involved in Group 3A. Both TN and NC joints are involved in Groups 3B and 3C. Group 3B, with TN > NC affection, has the highest incidence of Maceira stage V. Group 3C, also termed reverse Müller-Weiss disease, with NC > TN involvement has the greatest second metatarsal overlength and midfoot abduction. Combining Wong groups and Maceira stages should elucidate geographical differences in disease pattern and provide a common reporting platform towards achieving gold standards of treatment.

**Keywords** Müller-Weiss disease · Maceira's classification · Méary's angle · Müller-Weissoid disease · Reverse Müller-Weissoid disease · Midfoot abduction

## Introduction

Any classification of a disease or condition should serve as guide to cause, treatment and prognosis. The classification introduced two decades ago by Maceira and Rochera is based solely on Méary's angle (Maceira et al. 2004). Although it describes pathomechanics, it does not guide treatment or prognosis. As a result, there is no set gold standard for the operative or nonoperative management of Müller-Weiss disease.

© The Author(s), under exclusive license to Springer Nature Switzerland AG 2024 
J. Wong-Chung, *Comprehensive Guide to Müller-Weiss Disease*,
https://doi.org/10.1007/978-3-031-66644-5_4

This Chapter discusses Maceira's classification and attempts to modify it. It also expounds upon the recently proposed grouping system by Wong-Chung et al. in 2023 (2023).

## 4.1 Classification Incorporating Pathomechanics by Maceira and Rochera, 2004

The only classification of Müller-Weiss disease in current usage is that propounded by Maceira and Rochera in 2004 (Fig. 4.1). It is based solely on Méary's talo-first metatarsal angle as measured on lateral weight-bearing radiographs of the foot and ankle (Maceira and Rochera 2004).

### *4.1.1 Stage I*

In Stage I, plain radiographs show minimal or no bony changes while scintigraphy detects increased activity and MRI demonstrates bone marrow oedema. Méary's angle is normal, but subtle heel varus is present. Of the 191 feet in Maceira and Rochera's series, 19% were at Stage I. These were usually feet on the less affected side in bilateral disease.

### *4.1.2 Stage II*

A short first metatarsal produces a lateral shift of compressive forces. Suboptimal ossification, caused by nutritional or environmental factors, weakens the navicular chondral anlage rendering it more vulnerable to abnormal stresses. Flattening and deformity of the lateral navicular ensues. Using three-dimensional computed tomography, Maceira and Rochera demonstrated compression and flattening of the posterior surface of the lateral half of the navicular. They likened the resultant bone to 'squeezed plastic material' in the shape of a comma or hourglass.

With compression of the lateral portion of the navicular, the talar head displaces laterally and dorsalward to lie over the anterior process of the calcaneus instead of beside it. Radiography demonstrates dorsal rotatory subluxation of the talar head and Méary's angle changes to apex dorsal in Stage II. Since the calcaneum forms part of the 'acetabulum pedis', it follows by moving into varus, as the talar head shifts lateralward. Subtalar varus increases and radiological signs of subtalar inversion are evident, namely an open sinus tarsi and an elongated cyma S line implying decreased superimposition of the talar head upon the anterior calcaneal process (Figs. 4.1, 4.2). Of the 191 feet, 9% were at Stage II.

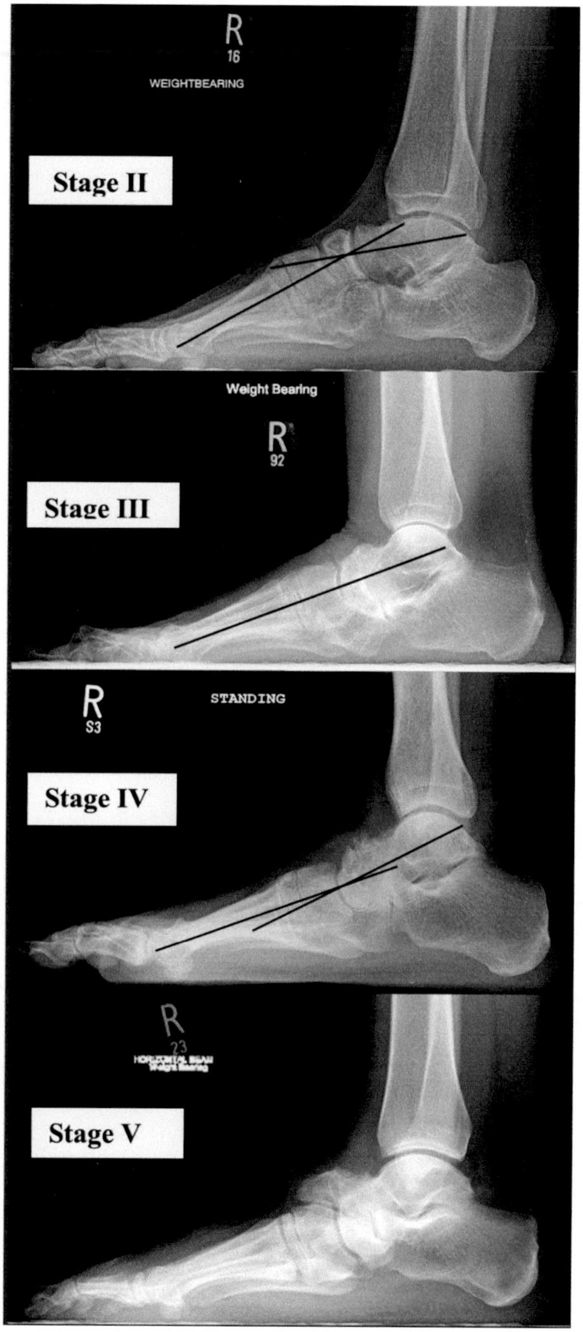


**Fig. 4.1** Maceira and Rochera's Stages. An apex dorsal Méary's angle in Stage II disease, dorsal rotatory subluxation of the talus, an elongated cyma line and a see-through sinus tarsi are indicative of subtalar varus. With further compression, the arch returns to neutral in Stage III and sags in Stage IV. The lateral navicular fragment extrudes dorsally in Stage V Müller-Weiss disease with the talar head articulating directly with the lateral cuneiform bone

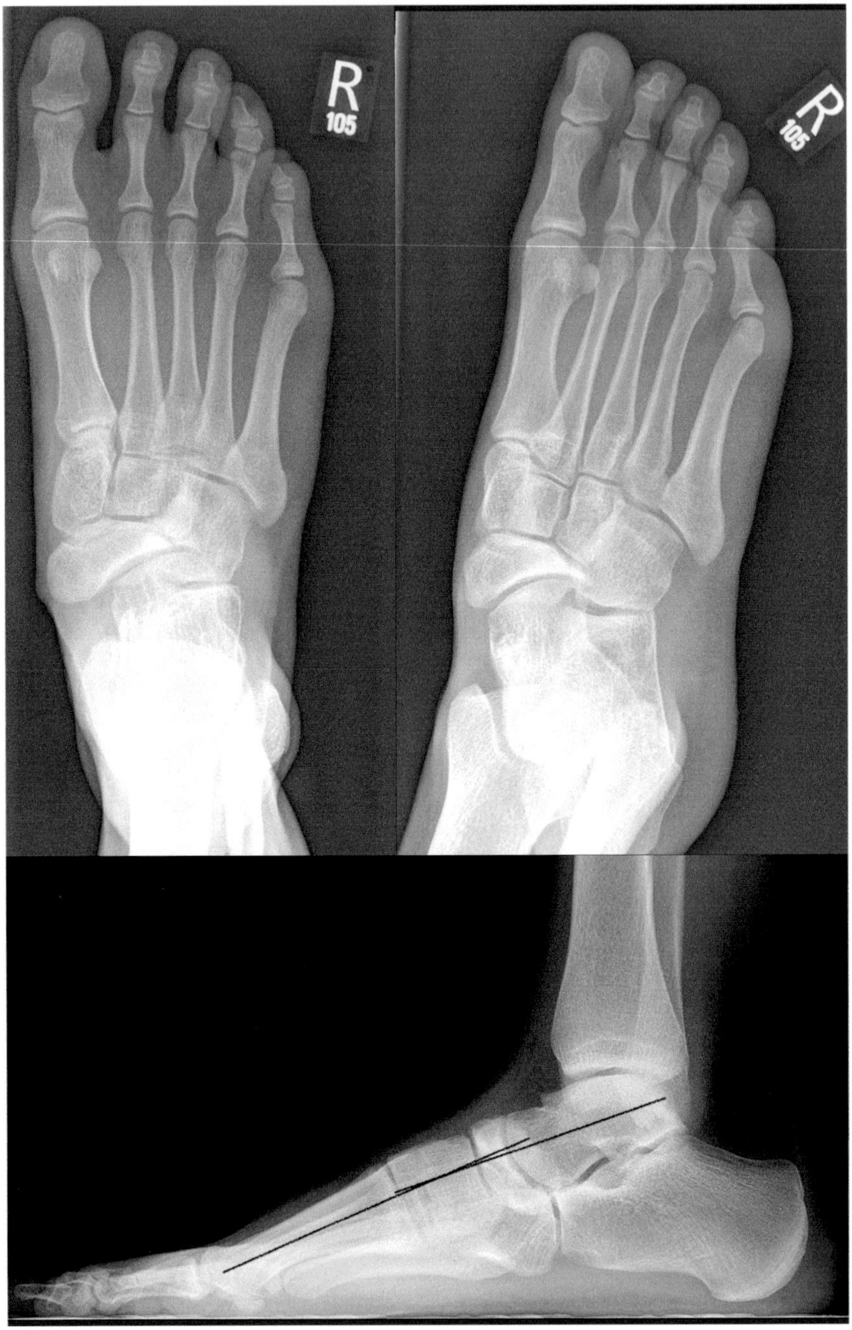
R
105
R
105

◂**Fig. 4.2** Dorsoplantar standing, medial oblique and lateral standing radiographs of the right foot of a 16-year-old boy demonstrating compression and fragmentation of the lateral navicular. Medial talonavicular subluxation with lateral shift of talar head. Méary's angle is positive indicating a Maceira Stage II. The middle and posterior facets of the subtalar joint and sinus tarsi are clearly visible. Elongated '*S*' shaped cyma line indicates decreased superimposition of talar head and anterior calcaneal process. The fracture line runs from dorsal distal to plantar proximal. Note also retropositioning of the fibular and decreased calcaneal pitch

As the disease evolves, compression increases and fragmentation of the lateral navicular ensues. A sagittal cleft develops in the navicular running from dorsal distal to plantar proximal at the level of the intermediate and lateral cuneiform bones (Fig. 4.2). Further splitting divides the navicular into a bigger medial portion and a smaller lateral or dorsolateral fragment.

### 4.1.3 Stage III

As compression and flattening extend to the lateral and plantar aspect of the navicular, the talar head shifts not only laterally but also plantarwards over the calcaneum, purportedly driving the hindfoot into equinus and the subtalar joint further into varus. The medial longitudinal arch returns to neutral in Stage III (46%).

### 4.1.4 Stage IV

In Stage IV disease, the medial arch starts to sag (19%) (Fig. 4.1). It does so due to failure of the beam component and not of the truss mechanism as in progressive collapsing foot deformity (PCFD). Signs of hindfoot varus are present despite the fallen arch, hence the term 'paradoxical pes planus varus'.

### 4.1.5 Stage V

Degree of sagging increases with progressive compression, collapse and fragmentation of the navicular. It reaches maximum value in end-stage V disease (7%), when the dorsolateral navicular fragment extrudes dorsally. With the medial navicular fragment subluxed medially enough, a space forms for the talar head to shift more laterally and inferiorly, driving the subtalar joint further into varus and squeezing the medial pole of the navicular even more medially. The plantarflexed and laterally displaced talar head articulates directly with the lateral cuneiform bone, forming the 'talo-cuneiform' articulation that characterizes Stage V disease (Figs. 4.1, 4.3). All the while, the heel is still in varus—the 'paradoxical pes planus varus'.

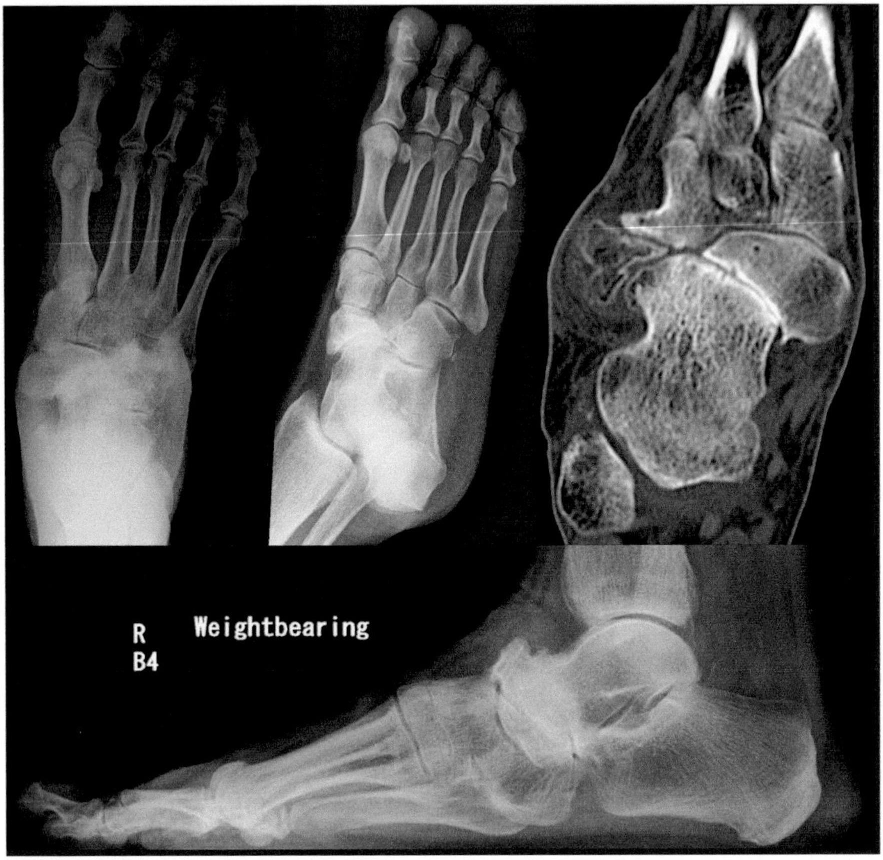


**Fig. 4.3** Example of Group 3B Maceira Stage V disease in a 62-year-old woman. The talonavicular is more affected than the naviculocuneiform joint. Fragmentation of the lateral navicular with dorsal extrusion of the lateral navicular fragment and medial arch sag. Medial talonavicular subluxation and lateral shift of the talar head. Broken cyma lines. End-stage V disease is marked by the talocuneiform articulation, the talar head articulating directly with the lateral cuneiform bone, as confirmed on CT scan

It is important to note that the navicular bone is not being squeezed out such that it 'extrudes' medially per se. Apparent medial extrusion of the medial pole of the navicular is due to medial talonavicular subluxation, as the talar head also moves laterally and inferiorly.

### 4.1.6 *Remarks by Maceira and Rochera*

Maceira and Rochera remarked that the arch always sags in advanced PCFD with talonavicular arthritis. However, in Müller-Weiss disease, it is not surprising to encounter talonavicular arthritis with the arch well-maintained, presumably referring to Stages II and III.

Although they have recorded progression of compression and osteoarthritis during follow-up of their patients, they have not noticed transition from one stage of the disease to the next. Neither have they noticed a navicular that was intact go on to develop fragmentation. They therefore postulated that all five stages develop progressively during infancy while the navicular is still made up of chondral cartilage rather than bone. The children do not complain of pain, as the cartilage has no innervation. Once ossification resumes, deformity does not progress. However, any morphological and biomechanical changes that have already happened persist throughout the rest of the patient's life.

Maceira's classification thus describes increasing sag of the medial longitudinal arch with greater degrees of compression and fragmentation of the navicular. Importantly, the authors stressed that their staging system does not necessarily correlate with symptomatology. For example, a foot at Stage I may be very painful while symptoms in another foot at Stage IV or V may be manageable. However, they regard their staging system as a valuable tool for descriptive purposes. Monteagudo and Maceira later admitted that, while it may give some information about pathomechanics of the disease, it serves neither as guide to treatment nor prognosis (Monteagudo and Maceira 2019).

## 4.2 Proposed Modification by Mayich, 2016

Mayich (2016) lamented that Maceira's classification system did not clarify which joints are involved across the various stages (Mayich 2016). He considered involvement of the subtalar joint to be a distinguishing factor between Stages III and IV of the disease, as it is always involved in Stage IV.

He therefore proposed a modified Maceira classification with subtalar arthritis as a necessary criterion for diagnosis of Stage IV disease. In his experience, surgical intervention typically involved fusion of the talonavicular and naviculocuneiform joints. In Stage IV disease, additional subtalar arthrodesis would be indicated through which hindfoot varus can be concurrently corrected by incorporating a lateral closing wedge. Otherwise, the subtalar joint should be preferentially spared in Stage III disease.

## 4.3 Monteagudo and Maceira, 2019

Monteagudo and Maceira elaborated further on the theoretical pathogenetic pathways in the evolution of Müller-Weiss disease (Monteagudo and Maceira 2019). Based on their experience, they believed that the disease starts mostly in childhood with two factors necessary for its formation. Reiterating delayed ossification as the prime prerequisite, they named their first category an *epidemic* group consisting of the so-called "children of war", who had not been able to completely ossify their navicular bone due to environmental or nutritional stress. A necessary second factor is lateral displacement of compression forces caused by brachymetatarsia of the first ray. During the third rocker, axial compression forces are then transmitted mostly between the talar head and middle/lateral cuneiforms bone duo and produce plastic deformation of the lateral part of a navicular already weakened by delayed ossification. An immature navicular chondral anlage would be able to cope with compression stresses, if they were evenly distributed along its entire surface, as in Köhler's disease. It would also tolerate uneven compression well in a child with limited physical activities.

The previous statement introduces their second category, which is a "*non-epidemic'* group made up usually of athletes who had undergone intensive training during childhood. They bear no record of past environmental or nutritional stress, as evidenced by dental abnormalities and porosities on the outer table of the cranial vault or 'cribra orbitalia'. Despite navicular ossification having proceeded on schedule, it was subjected to "too much too soon." The first ray was also short in these children either because of real shortening of the first metatarsal or as a result of relative shortening of the medial column secondary to internal rotation of the navicular in the transverse plane and retroposition of TMT1 relative to TMT2.

The authors further contend that, beyond the scenario of a normally developing navicular in a child being subjected to mechanical forces expected in an adult, a subtle underlying condition may also exist to enable shifting of the talar head towards the lateral side of the coxa pedis, such as metatarsus adductus, either primary or as part of a subtle congenital talipes equinovarus, subtalar varus or both. Rochera had noticed delayed ossification of the navicular in children with metatarsus adductus. Spontaneous correction of forefoot adductus by "en-bloc" external rotation of the cuneiforms and cuboid has been observed. Such rotation is only possible through compression of the lateral part of the navicular and medial suluxation of the cuboid, the fulcrum being the medial aspect of the navicular. The mechanism can be likened to a 'nutcracker', with the talus and cuneiform bones representing the arms, the medial aspect of the navicular being the fulcrum and the nut being the lateral aspect of the navicular.

Their third category describes feet, in which the disease develops in a previously healthy adult navicular and are termed "Müller-Weissoid" feet. These may easily be mistaken for acquired flatfoot or progressive collapsing foot deformity, as the feet were previously normal. A combination of a short first metatarsal and subtalar varus is believed to play a role in development of this "adult-onset" Müller-Weiss disease by promoting pronation and abduction of the midfoot and forefoot.

## 4.4 Grouping System by Wong-Chung et al. (2023)

While Maceira's classification is based only on the lateral Méary's angle, the grouping system put forward by Wong-Chung et al. takes into account: (1) age of onset (2) previous evidence of a radiologically normal navicular (3) which perinavicular joints are affected (4) dorsoplantar talo-first metatarsal angle and (5) lateral Méary's angle (Wong-Chung et al. 2023). The authors recommend that future studies report outcomes of treatment according to a combination of their grouping system and Maceira's stages. Only through a common platform for reporting Müller-Weiss disease can gold standards in treatment be defined, which Maceira's classification does not presently allow.

Wong-Chung et al. (Northern Ireland, 2023) performed a detailed radiographic analysis of 95 feet in 37 female and 30 male patients. Firstly, the latest radiographs were scrutinized to ensure the feet met the minimum criteria for inclusion in the study, namely compression of the lateral portion of the navicular, medial extrusion of its medial pole, lateral shift of the talar head and resultant eccentric osteoarthrosis. Feet with concentric arthritis of the talonavicular joint did not have significant medial extrusion and were excluded from the study. Earliest radiographs were next examined for normality or presence of Müller-Weiss disease. On the first and each subsequent radiograph, the following were measured, including on the opposite foot in unilateral cases.

Measurements on dorsoplantar radiographs included anteroposterior thickness of the navicular at the midpoint of each naviculocuneiform joint, degree of medial extrusion of the navicular, Kite's anteroposterior talo-calcaneal angle, relative length of the second metatarsal with respect to the first and dorsoplantar talo-first metatarsal angle (See also Sect. 3.8). Presence and location of fracture were recorded. Sites and severity of osteoarthritis were graded according to Kellgren-Lawrence scale (1957) and intensity of radio-isotope uptake on SPECT-CT. Méary's angles, as measured on lateral weight-bearing radiographs, provided Maceira disease stages.

They identified 3 distinct groups, based on (1) age of onset (2) radiographic evidence of a previously normal navicular bone and talonavicular joint and (3) the joints affected. For each group, magnitude of compression and navicular extrusion, Kite's angle, dorsoplantar talo-first metatarsal angle and Méary's angle, metatarsal indices, presence of fracture and sites of osteoarthritis were analyzed.

### 4.4.1 Early-Onset Wong Group 1

The "early-onset" Group 1 comprised the 11 youngest feet, aged 9 to 29 (median, 22.7) years old at first presentation ($p < 0.001$). The condition was bilateral in all except 1. It had the greatest degree of compression at the level of the lateral naviculocuneiform joint, the greatest degree of medial extrusion ($p = 0.001$) and the lowest Kite's angle ($p < 0.001$). All had a fracture at the lateral corner of the navicular except one (Odds radio = 27.3) ($p < 0.001$). All were index minus except one. Early degeneration was seen in 3 older feet aged 31 to 33 years at last follow-up, and moderate changes at 1 talonavicular joint in a 32-year-old. None has undergone surgery so far, although a man now aged 29 years old presented recently with worsening symptoms severe enough that he wishes to proceed to surgery.

The postulated mechanism in the 'early-onset' feet is that an index minus metatarsal formula leads to compression of the young relatively soft navicular between the talar head and lateral/middle cuneiform bone duo. The lateral blood supply of the navicular is hence impaired. Fracture of the lateral corner ensues, allowing greater degree of medial subluxation of the talonavicular joint and apparent medial extrusion of the medial navicular pole. In turn, the medially subluxed navicular pushes the talar head further laterally with a resultant decrease in Kite's angle (Fig. 4.4).

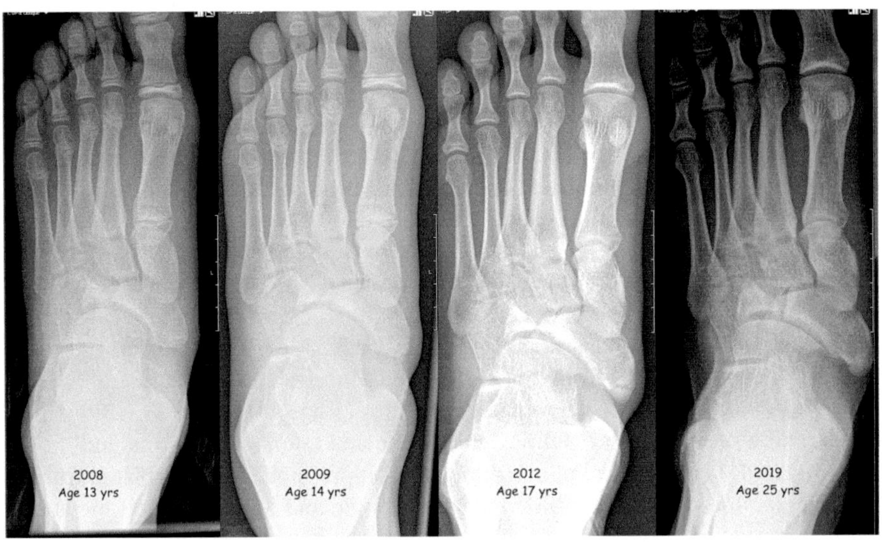


**Fig. 4.4** Serial dorsoplantar radiographs of a boy with early-onset Müller-Weiss disease. Overlong hypertrophied second metatarsal causes compression and fragmentation at the lateral corner of the navicular and medial extrusion. In turn, the medially subluxed navicular pushes the talar head further laterally with further decrease of Kite's angle. No radiological sign of osteoarthritis is visible 12 years later

### 4.4.2 *Late-Onset Wong Group 2 ≡ Müller-Weissoid Feet*

The second group corresponds to the "Müller-Weissoid" feet, as termed by Monteagudo and Maceira to describe feet which develop Müller-Weiss disease in late adulthood, having had previously normal naviculars at an unspecified age in early adulthood (Monteagudo and Maceira 2019). Twenty-three feet, aged 49 to 82 (median, 61) years old, had radiologically normal navicular 0.4 to 10.4 years earlier (median, 6.7; IQR, 5.7 to 7.4 years).

The "Müller-Weissoid" feet had the lowest degree of compression at both middle and lateral naviculocuneiform joints ($p = 0.002$), the lowest degree of medial extrusion and the highest Kite's angles. Not all were index minus with 6 of 23 feet being index positive. Overlength of the second relative to the first metatarsal was lower than in other groups. None had a complete fracture, except for one in which CT suggested an infraction but no fracture was visible at arthrodesis surgery (Fig. 4.5A–J). Degeneration occurred at the talonavicular joint in all cases. Additional early asymptomatic changes were seen at the lateral naviculocuneiform joint in 10 and moderate changes at both middle and lateral naviculocuneiform joints in 1 foot.

Since the navicular bone was previously normal well into the sixth decade of life, the authors postulate that development of Müller-Weiss disease in these feet is primarily an arthritic process resulting from prolonged repetitive asymmetrical compression of the hyaline cartilage of the navicular.

### 4.4.3 *Late-Onset Wong Group 3*

Patients in the third group were first diagnosed with Müller-Weiss disease in adulthood, on average in their sixth decade, and had no previous documentation of a radiologically normal navicular. This 'late-onset' group is further subdivided into 3 subgroups according to which joints are involved.

With any of the groups and subgroups, the subtalar ± calcaneocuboid joints may or may not also be involved. Unlike Mayich whose focus was on the subtalar joint, Wong-Chung et al.'s grouping system distinguishes between involvement of the talonavicular joint only and affection of both talonavicular and naviculocuneiform joints, especially in Group 3.

#### Late-Onset Wong Group 3A

Excluding the subtalar and calcaneocuboid articulations, Group 3A affects the talonavicular joint only (Fig. 4.6A–I).

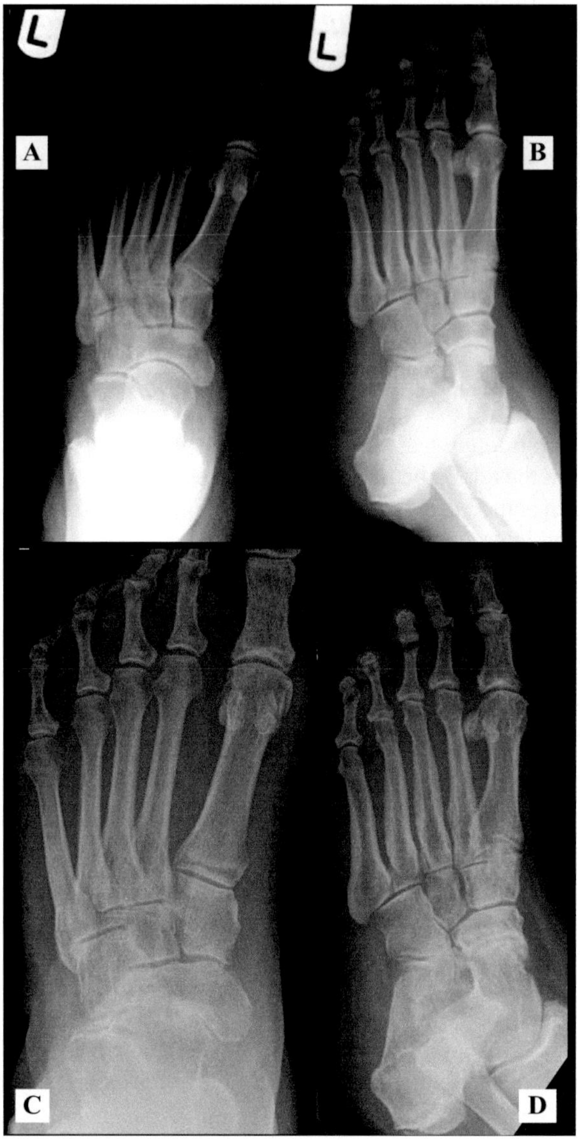


**Fig. 4.5** Case of Müller-Weissoid disease in a 61-year-old woman. (A) Dorsoplantar and (B) medial radiographs of the left foot showing a normal navicular. The second metatarsal is slightly longer than the first. (C) Dorsoplantar standing and (D) medial oblique views 3 years later reveal a comma-shaped navicular with compression of its lateral part and advanced arthritis at the talonavicular joint. CT images demonstrate advanced talonavicular arthritis with osteophyte formation at the anterior facet of the subtalar joint and 4-corners. The lateral naviculocuneiform (NC3) joint is not affected. A fracture line is seen at the level of the lateral cuneiform on (E) axial and (F) coronal slices running distally and laterally towards the lateral corner of NC3. It is not visualized on any of the (G) sagittal slices. Nor could any fracture line be seen at surgery. (H-J) Triple arthrodesis fixed with a retrograde Arthrex 6.7 mm screw (Arthrex Inc, Naples, FL) across the subtalar joint and Uni-Clips across the talonavicular and calcaneocuboid joints (Integra Life Sciences, Plainsboro, NJ)

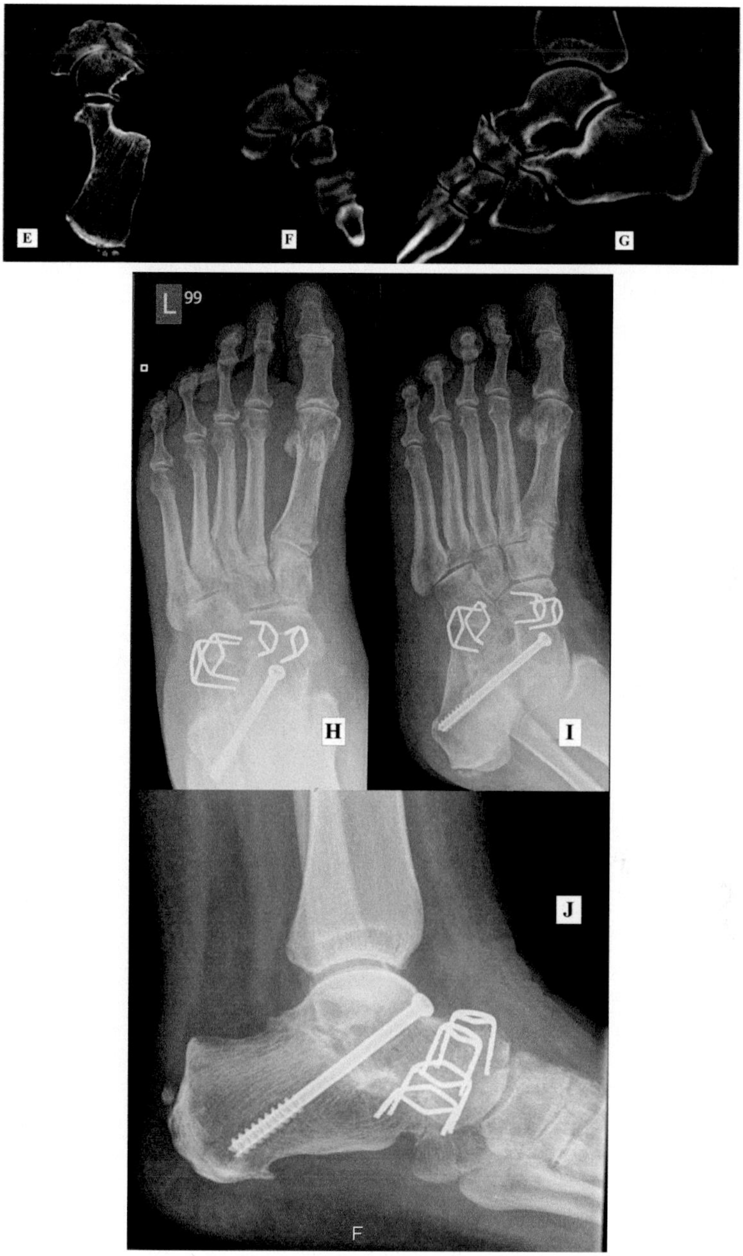


**Fig. 4.5** (continued)

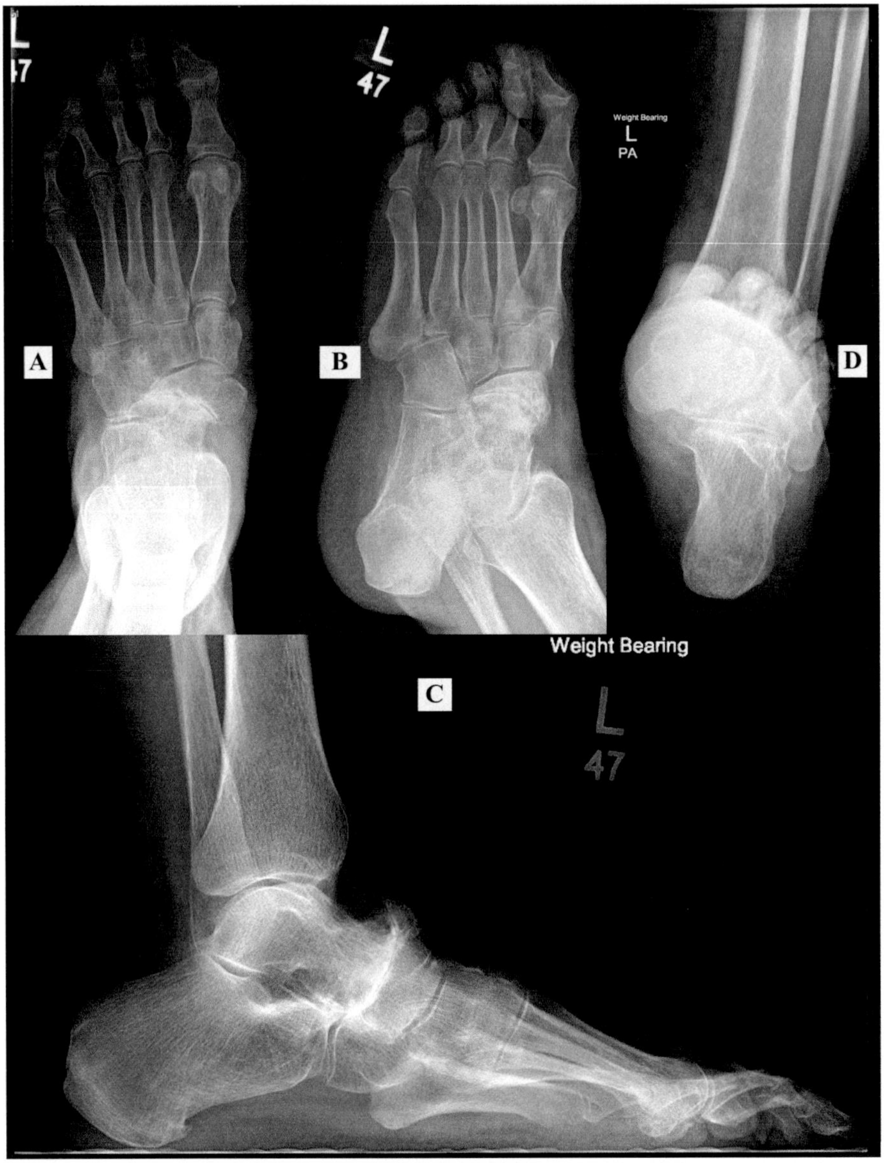


**Fig. 4.6** (A) Dorsoplantar standing radiograph of the left foot demonstrating Group 3A disease affecting the talonavicular joint. Compression of the lateral navicular with medial extrusion. Second metatarsal is longer than the first. Naviculocuneiform joints appear intact on (B) medial oblique view. (C) Normal Méary's angle on (C) lateral standing of left foot and ankle. Neutral heel position on (D) hindfoot alignment view. SPECT-CT reveals marked radioisotope uptake at the talonavicular joint on (E) coronal images. (F) Sagittal slice demonstrates mild to moderate degeneration and uptake at the 4-corners and anterior facet of the subtalar joint. Intact and quiescent naviculocuneiform joints. (G-I) Double medial arthrodesis fixed with retrograde Arthrex 6.7 mm screw (Arthrex Inc, Naples, FL) across the subtalar joint and 2 Uni-CP compression plates across the talonavicular joint (Integra Life Sciences, Plainsboro, NJ)

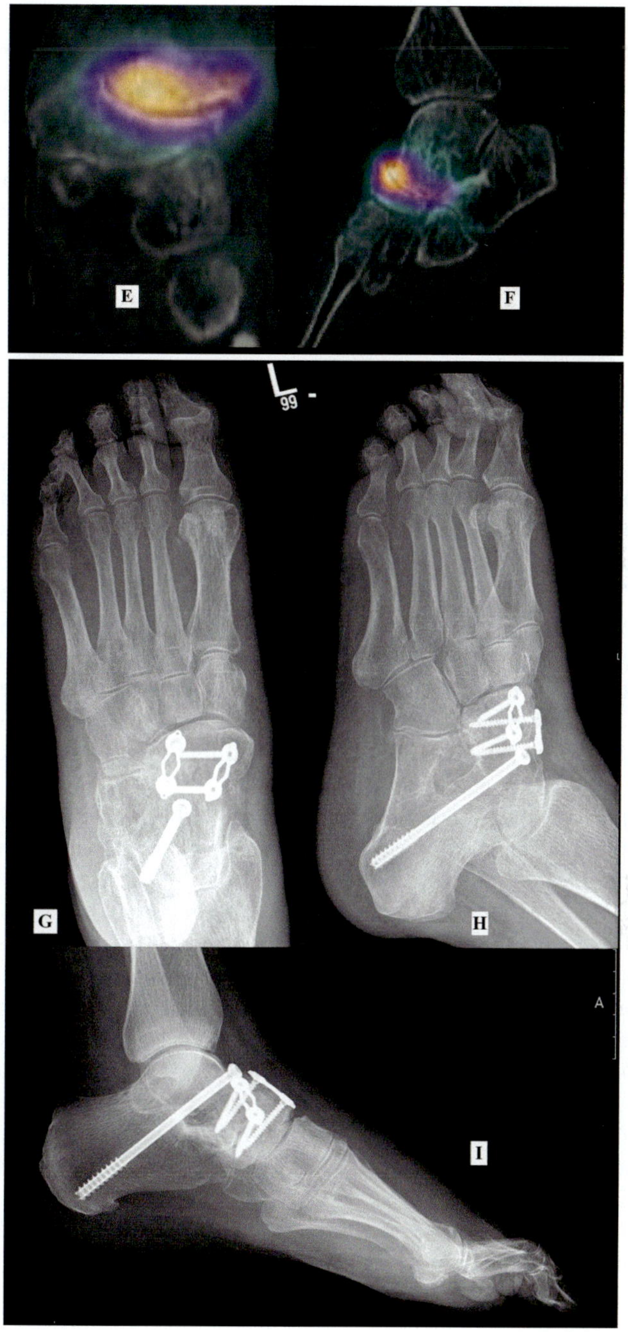


**Fig. 4.6** (continued)

### Late-Onset Wong Group 3B

Both talonavicular and naviculocuneiform joints are affected in Groups 3B and 3C.

Group 3B, in which the talonavicular joint is more predominantly affected than the naviculocuneiform joint, has the highest incidence of Maceira Stage V disease whereby the talar head articulates directly with the lateral cuneiform bone following fragmentation and dorsal extrusion of the lateral navicular fragment ($p = 0.001$) (Fig. 4.7A–Q).

### Late-Onset Wong Group 3C

Group 3C feet are also termed “reverse Müller-Weiss”, because compression is mostly at the naviculocuneiform side rather than at the talonavicular side. In their original account, Maceira and Rochera had described compression of the posterior surface of the navicular, despite their cadaveric specimen clearly showing more compression on the naviculocuneiform side. Various subsequent radiographic examples in the literature, including those of Monteagudo and Maceira, have also shown compression predominantly on the naviculocuneiform rather than on the talonavicular side. The authors postulate that many cases get labelled as Müller-Weiss disease at first glance, because what is immediately apparent on radiographs to the observer is compression of the lateral part of the navicular. But, upon closer look, one can then discern that in some cases, compression is on the talonavicular side as in the original description by Maceira and Rochera, and that in other cases, compression is more marked on the naviculocuneiform side.

For example, compression is clearly shown to be more marked at the naviculocuneiform rather than at the talonavicular side on the plain radiograph and schematic diagram in the third column of the sixth illustration by Maceira and his co-author Rochera, (2004) in the fourth illustration with co-author Fernández de Retana in 2004, (Fernández de Retana et al. 2004) and in the first diagram and fourth illustration with co-author Monteagudo in 2019 (Monteagudo and Maceira 2019).

Throughout the literature, examples of bilateral cases are shown with both feet at different Maceira stages and belonging to different Wong groups. Figure 4.8 depicts such a case of bilateral disease in a man who underwent a right triple arthrodesis at the age of 64 years old for Group 3A disease affecting the subtalar and talonavicular joint only (Fig. 4.9A–B). Seven years later, a left talonaviculocuneiform arthrodesis was performed for Group 3C reverse Müller-Weiss disease with marked midfoot abduction (Fig. 4.10A–B).

This group had the highest degree of midfoot abduction as measured by the talo-first metatarsal angle on dorsoplantar standing radiographs ($p = 0.001$). It also had the greatest overlength of the second metatarsal relative to the first ($p = 0.002$).

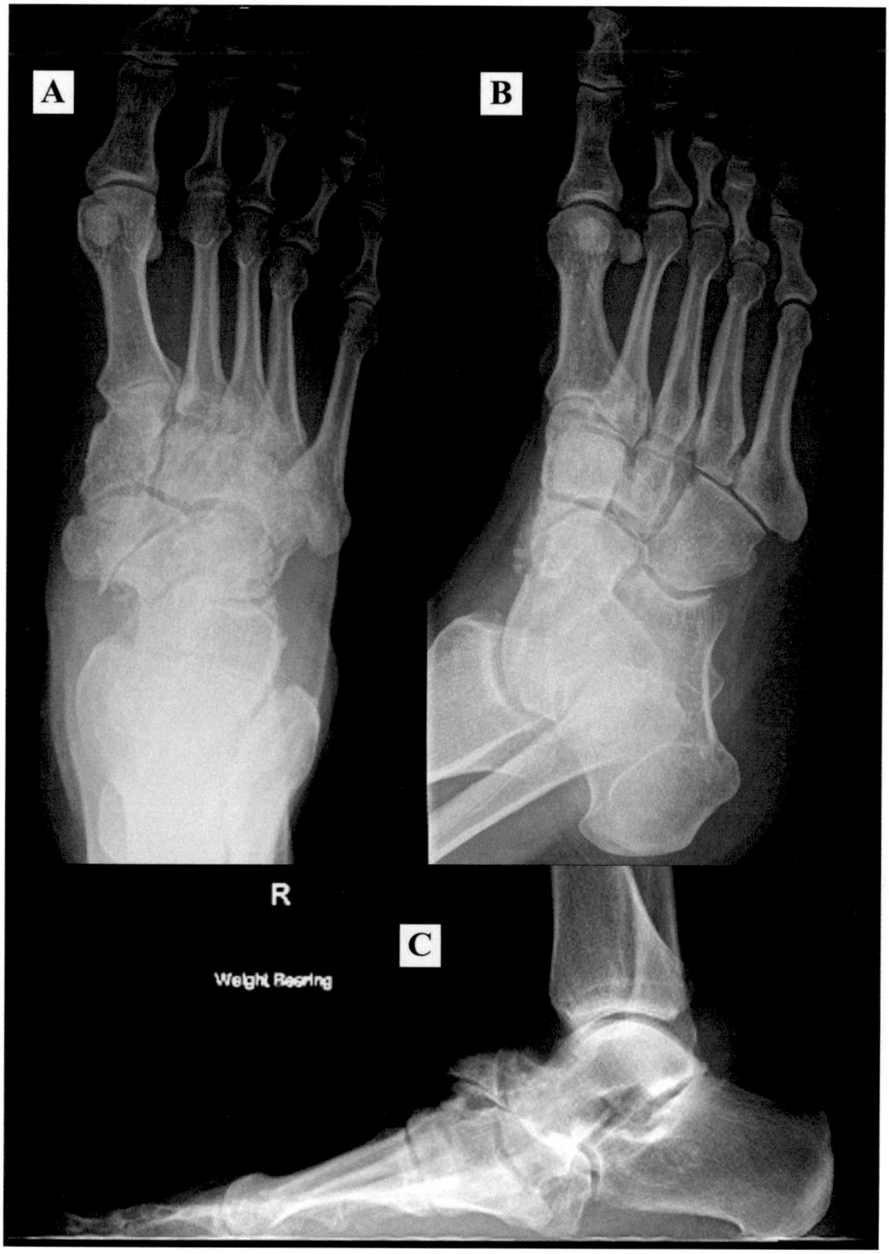
A
B
R
C
Weight Bearing

◀**Fig. 4.7** Group 3B Maceira Stage V disease. (A) Dorsoplantar standing radiograph shows severe compression of the lateral navicular and marked medial talonavicular subluxation with arthritis more advanced at the talonavicular than the naviculocuneiform joint. Direct articulation of the talar head with the lateral cuneiform bone on (B) medial oblique view. Dorsal extrusion of the lateral navicular fragment, sagging of the medial arch and plantar prominence formed by cuboid on (C) lateral standing radiograph of the foot and ankle. SPECT-CT. (D–G) Coronal and (H–K) sagittal images showing marked isotope uptake at an arthritic talonavicular joint. (F) Arthritic lateral naviculocuneiform and (G), (H) talocuneiform articulation. Intra-operative photographs depicting (I) dorsally extruded navicular fragment (M) excised and (N) advanced underlying talonavicular arthritis. (O–Q) Talonaviculocuneiform arthrodesis with interpositional tricortical iliac crest bone graft. Fixation with a proximal arch medial column locking plate and 2 dorsal bridging universal $2^8$ locking plates (Paragon 28, Englewood, CO). Medial arch sag has been corrected and the cuboid plantar prominence is less marked

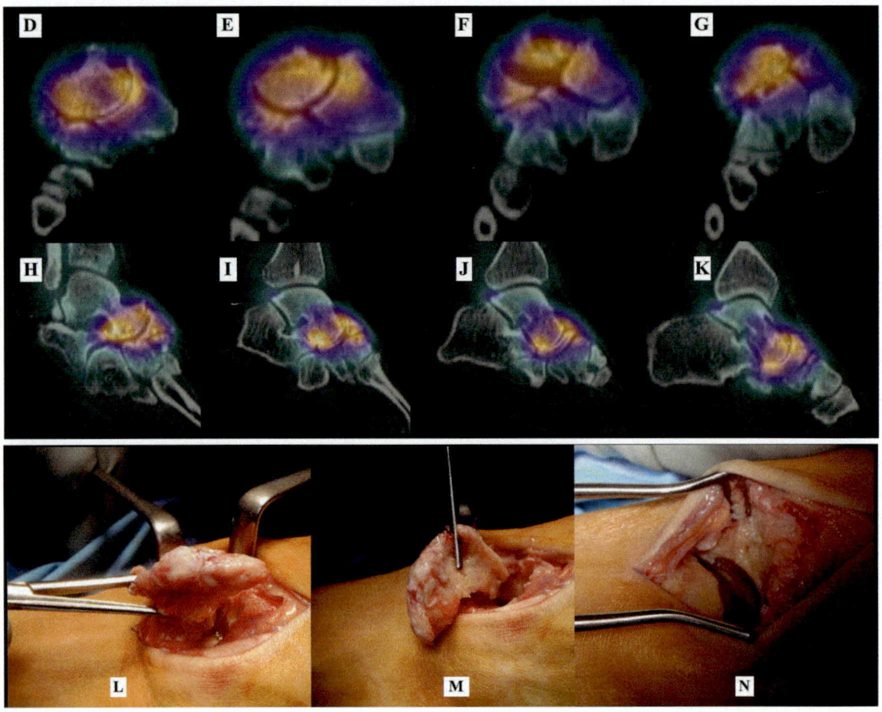


**Fig. 4.7** (continued)

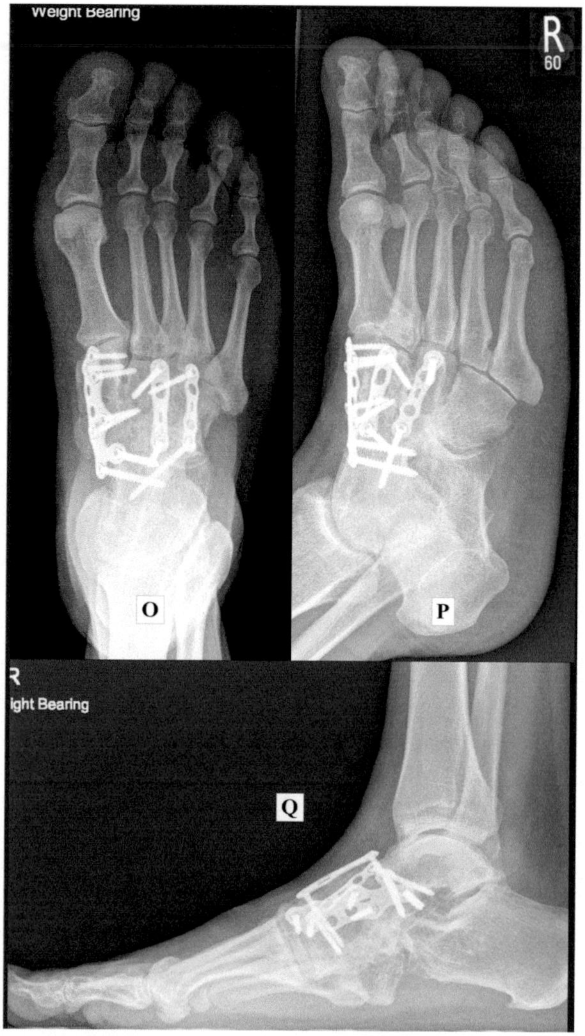


**Fig. 4.7** (continued)

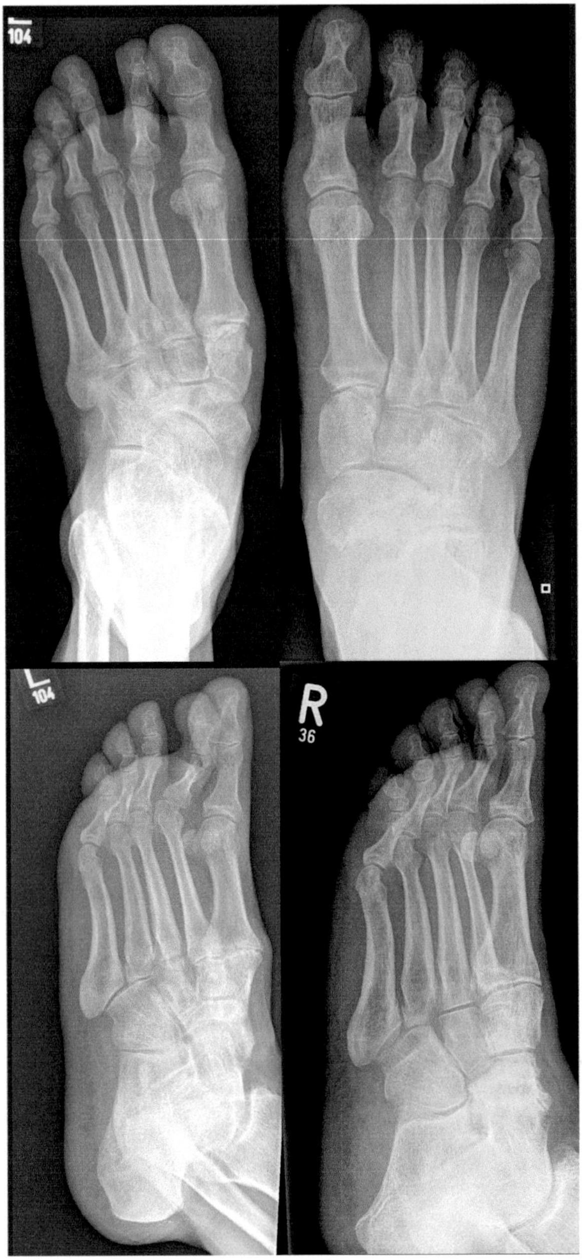


**Fig. 4.8** Different patterns of disease in a bilateral case. Group 3A affecting the right talonavicular joint and Group 3C reverse Müller-Weiss disease with compression of the left navicular more so on the naviculocuneiform than the talonavicular side

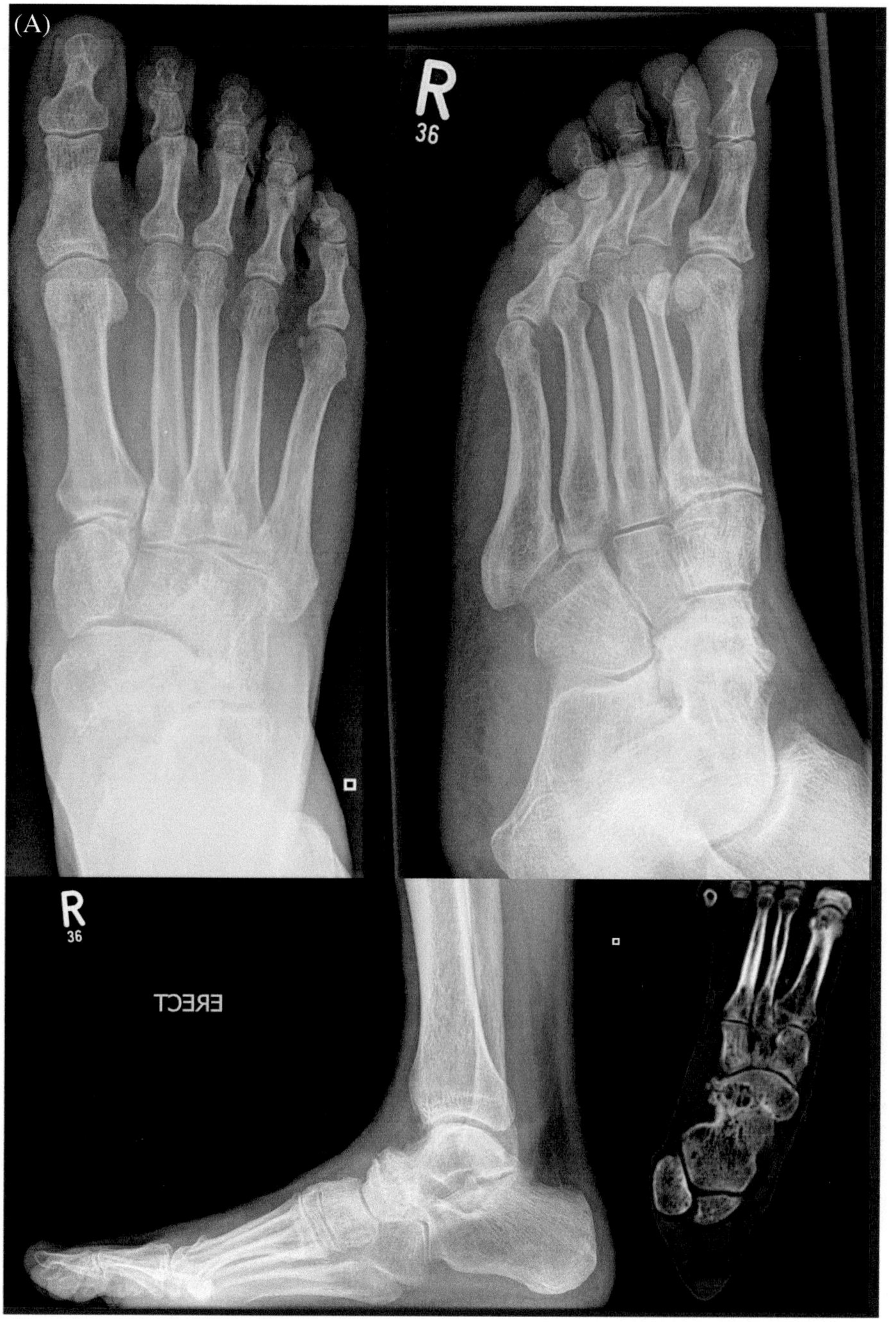


**Fig. 4.9** (A) Group 3A disease affecting the right talonavicular joint. The naviculocuneiform joint is intact according to CT scan. (B) Group 3A disease of the right foot treated by triple arthrodesis at age of 64 years old. Fixation with retrograde Arthrex 6.7 mm screw (Arthrex Inc, Naples, FL) across the subtalar joint and 2 Uni-CP compression plates across the talonavicular and 1 Uni-CP and 1 UniClip across the calcaneocuboid joint (Integra Life Sciences, Plainsboro, NJ)

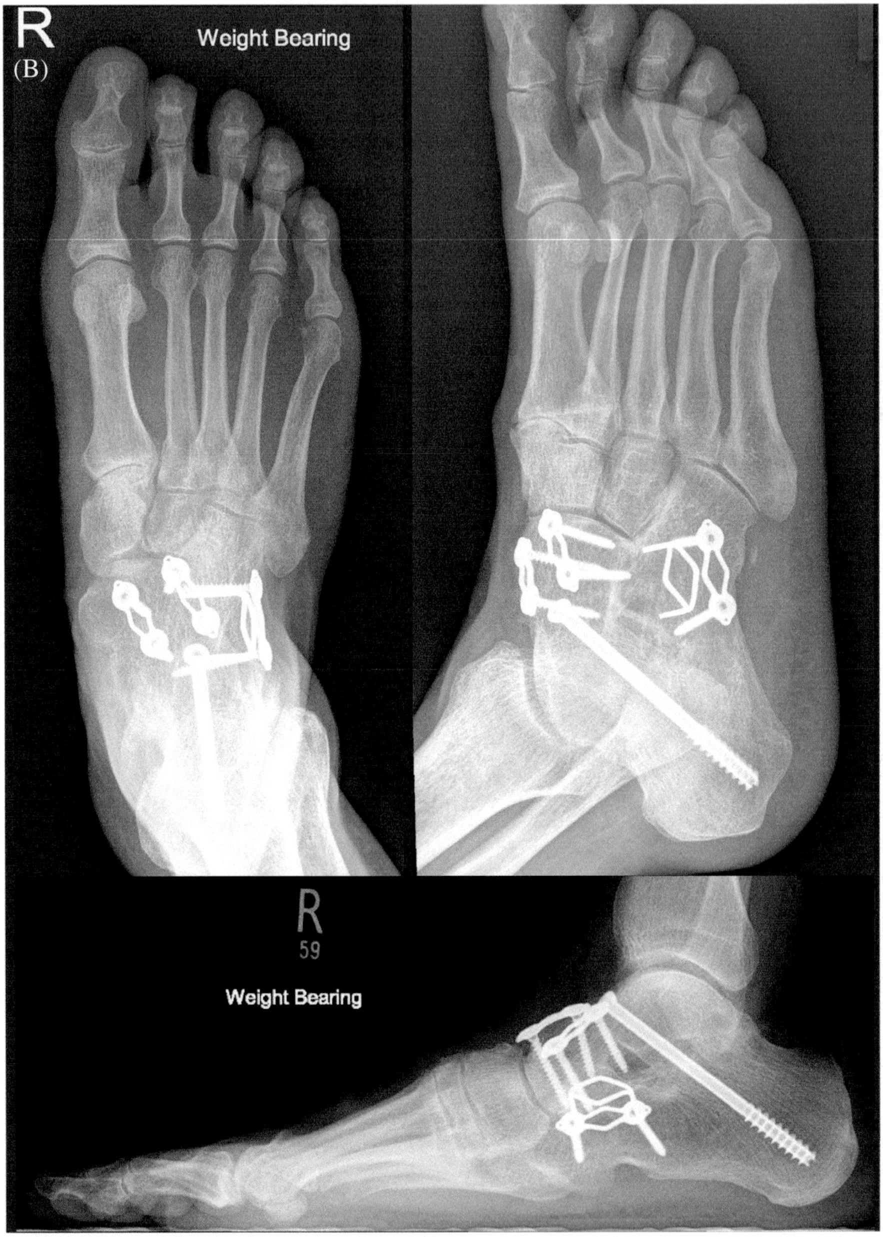


**Fig. 4.9** (continued)

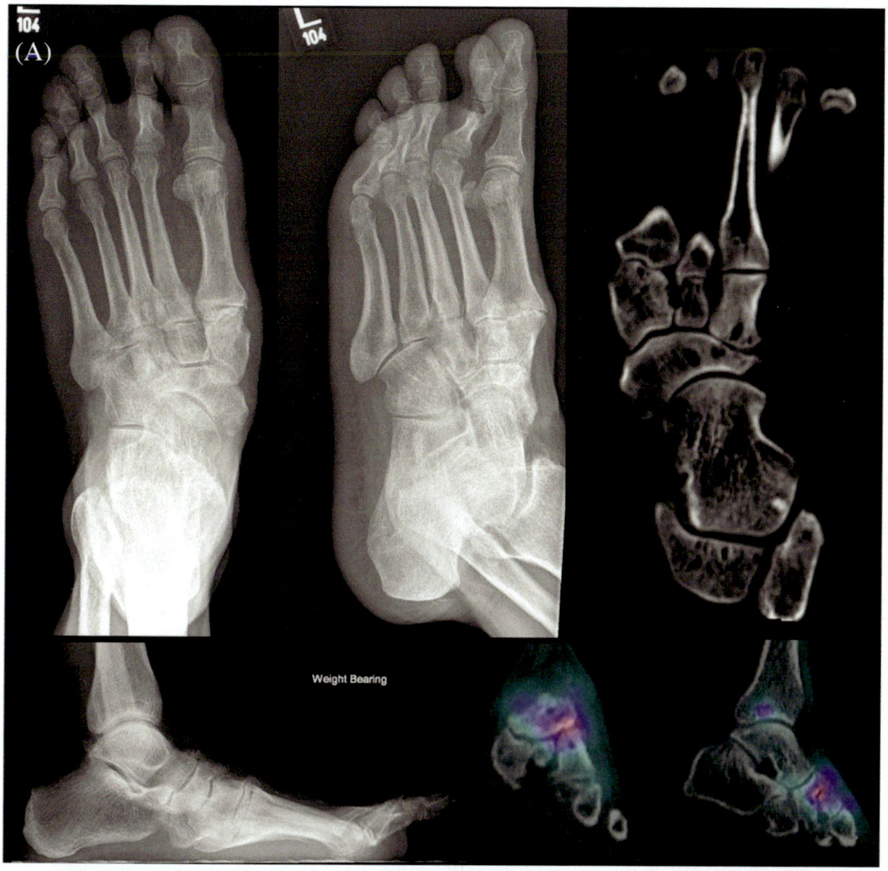


**Fig. 4.10** (A) The opposite left foot has Group 3C Maceira Stage IV reverse Müller-Weiss disease with compression and degenerative changes more marked on the naviculocuneiform side as evidenced by CT and SPECT-CT images. Dorsal osteophytes are more pronounced at the naviculocuneiform than at the talonavicular and tarsometatarsal joints. Marked midfoot abduction with dorsoplantar talo-first metatarsal angles of −35°. Second metatarsal is significantly longer than the first. Degenerative changes are also present at the first and second tarsometatarsal joints. Correction of left Group 3C reverse Müller-Weiss disease 7 years later by talonaviculocuneiform and tarsometatarsal (TMT) arthrodesis. Cancellous allograft bone chips packed at the lateral naviculocuneiform and TMT3 joints. Fixation with an arch medial column locking plate, dorsal locking universal $2^8$ across the second ray (Paragon 28, Englewood, CO) and a 2-hole Uni-CP plate across TMT3 (Integra Life Sciences, Plainsboro, NJ). Residual dorsiflexion at tarsometarsal level

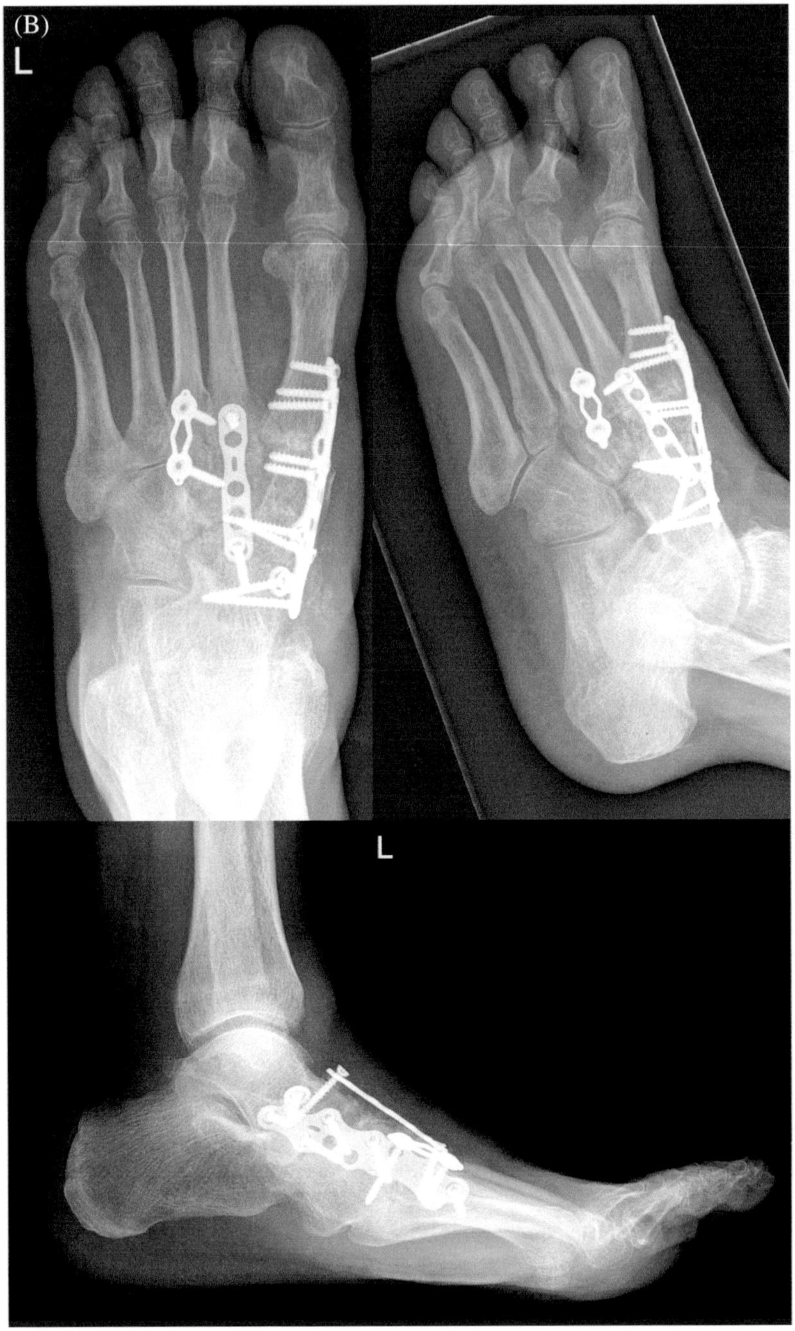


**Fig. 4.10** (continued)

**Characteristics of Wong Group 3**

All the Group 3C, all except one of Group 3A and 70% of Group 3B had an index minus metatarsal formula.

More compression occurs at the middle and lateral naviculocuneiform joints in Groups 3B and 3C than in 3A. No great difference exists in age distribution, degree of extrusion and Kite's angle among the late-onset Groups 3A, 3B and 3C.

No foot sustained a complete fracture in Group 3A. Incidence of fracture was 65% in Group 3B compared to 32% in Group 3C (Odds ratio = 4.6) ($p = 0.018$). When fracture occurs, degeneration also increases on the other less compressed side of the navicular bone.

## 4.5 No Correlation Between Medial Arch Sag and Navicular Compression

Taking all groups into account, no correlation was found between lateral Méary's angle and severity of navicular compression either at the middle ($p = 0.087$) or lateral ($p = 0.171$) naviculocuneiform joints. Degree of medial arch sag in Stage V disease is no greater than in Stage IV ($p = 0.351$). In fact, 3 feet with Stage V disease had notably raised medial arches, which would have been the expected findings in Stage II, when compression is meant to just start taking place, instead of Stage V. These findings invalidate Maceira's hypothesis of greater sag of the medial arch with increasing severity of navicular compression. Strong correlation existed between Méary's angle and the dorsoplantar talo-first metatarsal angles ($p < 0.001$).

## 4.6 A Reverse Müller-Weiss Pattern in the Egyptian Adolescent Feet

Ahmed et al. performed lateral column lengthening in 13 feet of 7 Egyptian adolescents aged 14 to 17 years old (Ahmed et al. 2019). While this approach may sound unconventional, scrutiny of their second set of illustrations reveals a Group 3C reverse Müller-Weiss pattern, in which the navicular is markedly more compressed on the naviculocuneiform side by an overlong second metatarsal, and 30° of midfoot abduction. Lateral column lengthening in their cases simultaneously corrected both sagging of the medial arch and the negative dorsoplantar talo-first metatarsal angle.

Medial extrusion of the medial navicular pole is still evident, although there does not appear to be significant medial subluxation at the talonavicular joint. The medial prominence is still formed by the navicular tuberosity and not the talar head. Kite's angle is decreased.

### 4.6.1 *Comparing Early-Onset Wong Group 1 with the Egyptian Adolescent Feet*

While the 11 feet with early-onset disease in the series of Wong-Chung et al. (2023) also showed compression more so on the naviculocuneiform than the talonavicular sides (Figs. 4.2, 4.4), midfoot abduction was not as marked with a median dorsoplantar talo-first metatarsal angle of + 1.73 degrees (IQR, −5.9 to 9). Instead, there was more marked medial talonavicular subluxation and a greater tendency to fragmentation at the lateral corner of the navicular. None has required surgery so far.

Ahmed et al. made no reference to occurrence of fracture in any of their 13 adolescent feet (Ahmed et al. 2019). Perhaps, fragmentation at the lateral corner of the navicular in 91% of the Northern Irish feet permitted more marked medial subluxation at the talonavicular joint, thereby dampening the amount of forefoot abduction caused by an overlong second ray. There may exist a geographical difference in pattern of the disease, which warrants further investigation.

## 4.7 Analysis of the Wong Group 2 Müller-Weissoid Feet

In their series comprising 95 feet, Wong-Chung et al. (2023) found 23 that fitted Monteagudo and Maceira's *written* definition of "Müller-Weissoid", namely feet with radiologically normal navicular 'as young adults' that then went on to develop Müller-Weiss disease in later adulthood. They were aged 49 to 82 years old and had radiologically normal navicular 6.7 years earlier on average.

Monteagudo and Maceira disclosed neither the age of their patients nor the interval from normality to pathology (Monteagudo and Maceira 2019). They believed a short first metatarsal and subtalar varus contributed to development of disease in these feet. On the other hand, Wong-Chung et al. noted that not all their 23 "Müller-Weissoid" feet were index minus, 6 of them being index positive. Also, overlength of the second relative to the first metatarsal was lower than in all other groups. However, similar to the findings of Monteagudo and Maceira, none had a fracture except for one infraction.

Degeneration occurred mostly at the talonavicular joint in all cases of Wong-Chung et al. Additional early asymptomatic changes were noted at the lateral naviculocuneiform (NC) joint in 10 and moderate changes at both NC2 and NC3 in 1. Monteagudo and Maceira observed that arthritis commonly occurred in Müller-Weissoid feet, but exemplified with a different pattern (Wong-Chung et al. 2023). The case of bilateral disease in their fourth illustration shows some degree of mild compression of the lateral third of the navicular in 1981, more so on the right side. Compression is on the naviculocuneiform (NC) rather than on the talonavicular (TN) side. The second metatarsal is longer than the first. Bilateral bunions are present with hallux valgus angles of 40° and first inter-metatarsal angles of 14°. By 1994, arthritis had developed at both Lisfranc joints with midfoot abduction and pronation. Clinically, marked dorsomedial prominences of the midfoot gave pseudo appearances of flatfoot secondary to posterior tibial tendon dysfunction. The authors commented that arthritis at the Lisfranc joint may distract attention away from subluxation and degeneration at the perinavicular joint.

Analysis of the weight-bearing radiographs obtained in 1994 demonstrates progression of lateral navicular compression with osteoarthritis at both NC and TN joints bilaterally. On the left side, degenerative changes are maximal at the lateral and middle NC joints with lesser changes at the TN joint. On the right side, changes are again greater at the NC than at the TN joint. Degeneration at the right talonavicular joint is more pronounced than at the opposite left side. In both feet, the midfoot has drifted into marked abduction with negative dorsoplantar talo-first metatarsal (DPTFM) angles of -30º and established degeneration at the first tarsometatarsal (TMT1) joint, more marked on the left side with 'elephant's foot' appearances at the base of both first metatarsals. Hallux valgus appears to have resolved spontaneously on both sides. By contrast, the DPTFM angle averaged just + 0.5º in the 23 "Müller-Weissoid" feet of Wong-Chung et al.

Both feet shown in Monteagudo and Maceira's fourth illustration would be classed as Group 3C reverse Müller-Weiss disease, according to the grouping system of Wong-Chung et al. Because they started off as near normal, they could then be termed reverse Müller-Weissoid. In fact, 3 of the 95 feet of Wong-Chung et al. were designated as Group 3C "reverse Müller-Weissoid", because when normality changed to pathology 1.33, 7.5 and 14 years later, changes were more evident on the naviculocuneiform than the talonavicular side.

Figure 4.11 exemplifies such a case of a Group 3C "reverse Müller-Weissoid" foot in a 63-year-old woman. The navicular was radiologically normal in May 2007. The second metatarsal is hypertrophic and longer than the first. The second and third metatarsophalangeal joints are dislocated. Early changes are present at the first and second tarsometatarsal (TMT) joints. Repeat radiograph in August 2018, over 11 years later, show marked compression of the lateral navicular with degenerative changes more evident at the naviculocuneiform (NC) than at a minimally affected talonavicular joint. By May 2021, although arthritis is severe at the lateral third of the talonavicular joint, the medial two-thirds appear relatively well preserved as also seen on SPECT-CT (Fig. 4.12), whereas degeneration extends right across NC3-2-1. Arthritis at TMT1-2–3 has progressed. She underwent talonaviculocuneiform and TMT arthrodesis with correction of midfoot abduction (Fig. 4.13). Dislocation of the second and third metatarsophalangeal joints were asymptomatic and left alone. Dorsoplantar talo-first metatarsal angle measured −4º compared to −30º in Monteagudo and Maceira's patient. Otherwise, radiographic features in Fig. 4.11 are identical to those shown in the fourth illustration of Monteagudo and Maceira.

Earliest available radiograph of her opposite right foot in January 2020 already demonstrates features of a Group 3C reverse Müller-Weiss disease with changes more marked at the naviculocuneiform joint with relative sparing of the talonavicular joint (Fig. 4.14), as confirmed on SPECT-CT (Fig. 4.15). As with the left foot, the navicular

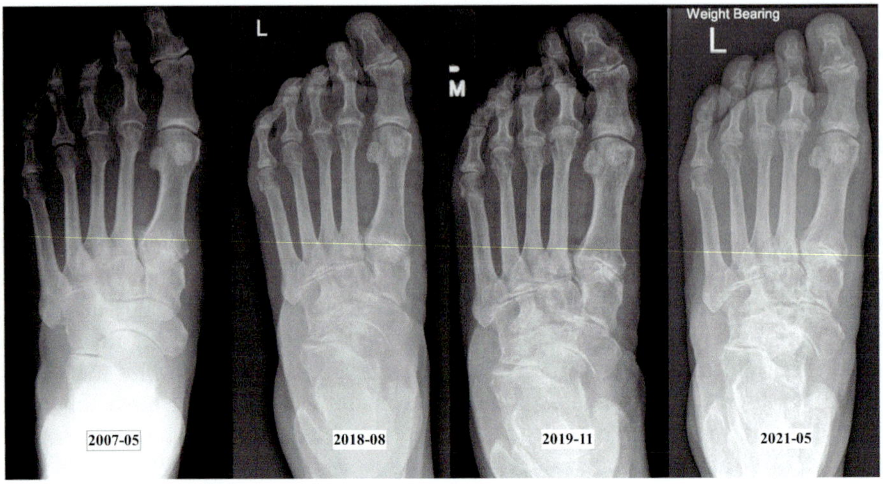


**Fig. 4.11** Reverse Müller-Weissoid disease in a 63-year-old woman whose navicular was radiologically normal in 2007. A hypertrophic second metatarsal is longer than the first. Dislocation of the second and third metatarsophalangeal joints. Early degeneration at the first and second tarsometatarsal (TMT) joints. Repeat radiograph in 2018 demonstrates marked compression of the lateral navicular with advanced degenerative changes at the naviculocuneiform (NC) joint. Mild narrowing and minor subchondral cyst formation at the lateral talonavicular joint space. Severe arthritis at the lateral third of the talonavicular joint in 2021. Its medial two-thirds appear relatively well preserved. Degeneration extends right across NC3-2-1. Arthritis at TMT1-2-3 has progressed

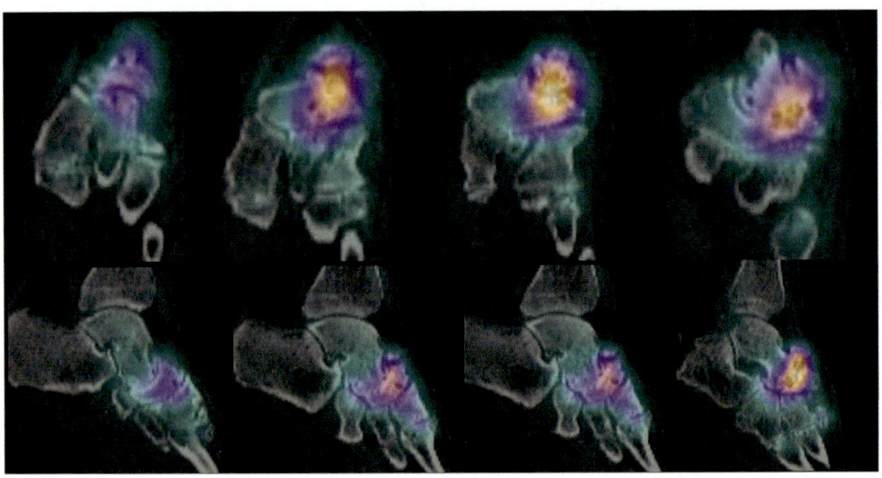

**Fig. 4.12** SPECT-CT coronal and sagittal images of the left foot

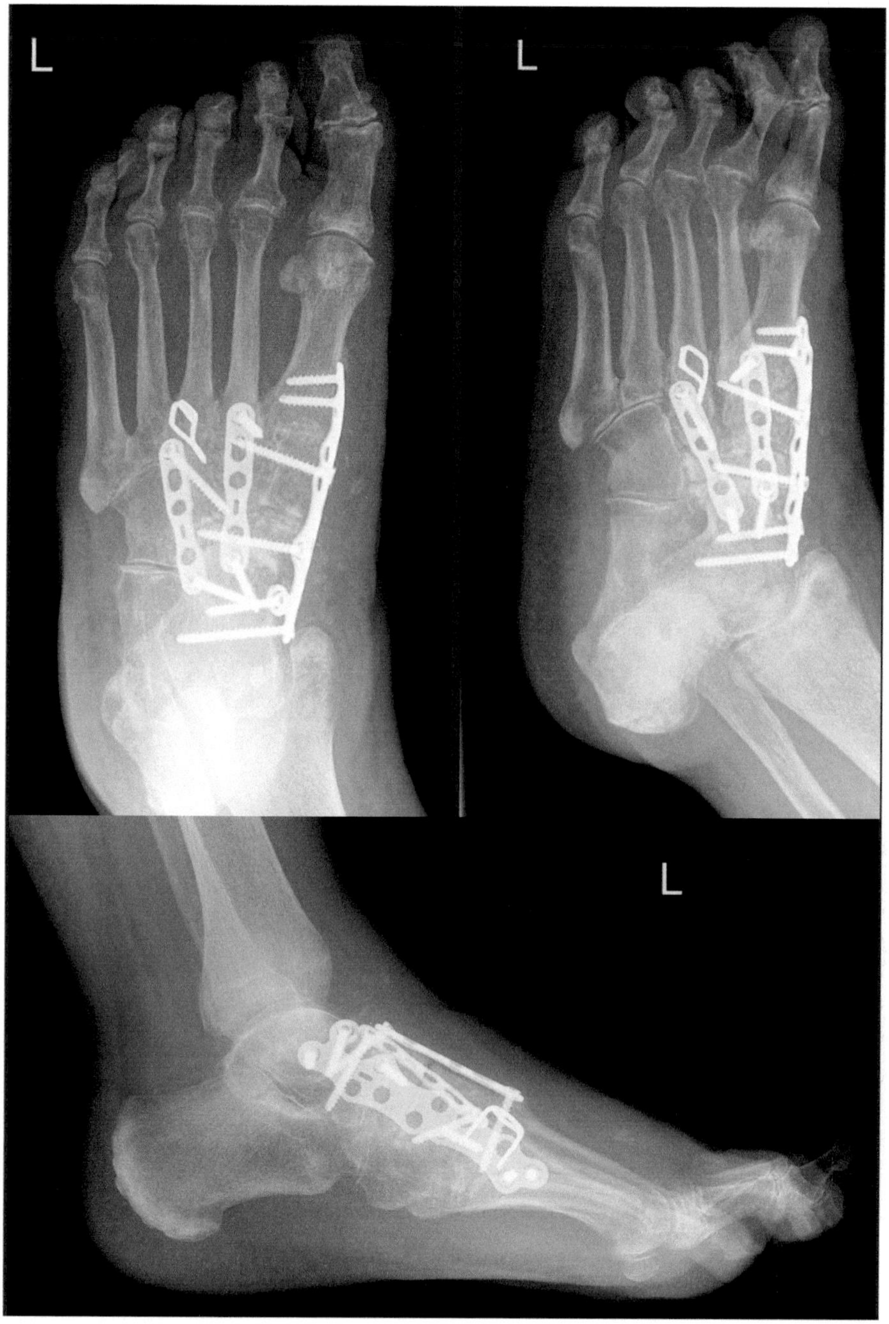


**Fig. 4.13** Postoperative radiographs following left talonaviculocuneiform arthrodesis extended to the tarsometatarsal (TMT) articulations. Fixation with an arch medial column plate, 2 dorsal $2^8$ universal locking plates (Paragon 28, Englewood, CO) and a UniClip staple across TMT3 (Integra Life Sciences, Plainsboro, NJ). For the second ray, the dorsal plate extends from the talar head to the base of the second metatarsal

may have shown up normal a decade earlier, had there been radiographs from that period.

In the other 2 “reverse Müller-Weissoid” feet, the earliest available radiographs already showed marked midfoot abduction with negative DPTFM angles of −18° and −37°, unlike Monteagudo and Maceira’s patient who exhibited DPTFM angles changing from positive to negative. It may be a question of having earlier radiographs, but then the other “reverse Müller-Weissoid” foot of Wong-Chung et al. had a negative DPTFM of just −4° fourteen years later.

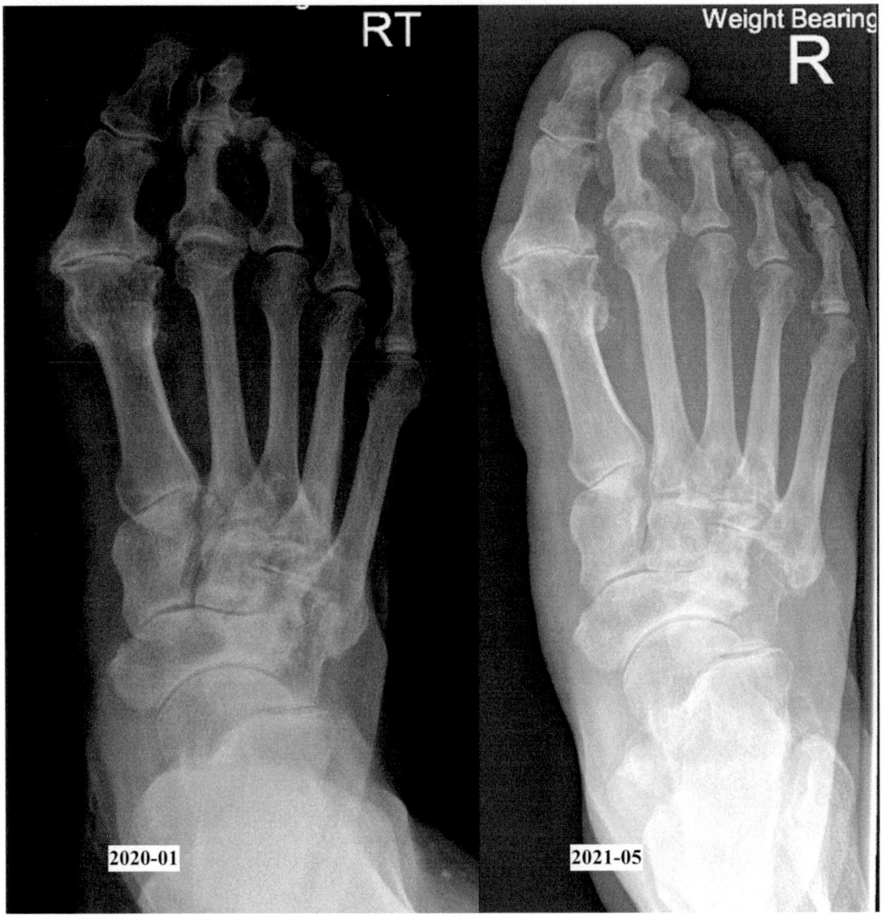


**Fig. 4.14** Earliest radiograph of the opposite asymptomatic right foot in January 2020 already shows compression and degenerative changes at the naviculocuneiform side with relative sparing of the talonavicular joint except for early lateral osteophyte formation and subchondral sclerosis. Arthritic first metatarsophalangeal (MTP) joint. Dislocated arthritic MTP2. Arthritis at TMT2 and TMT3

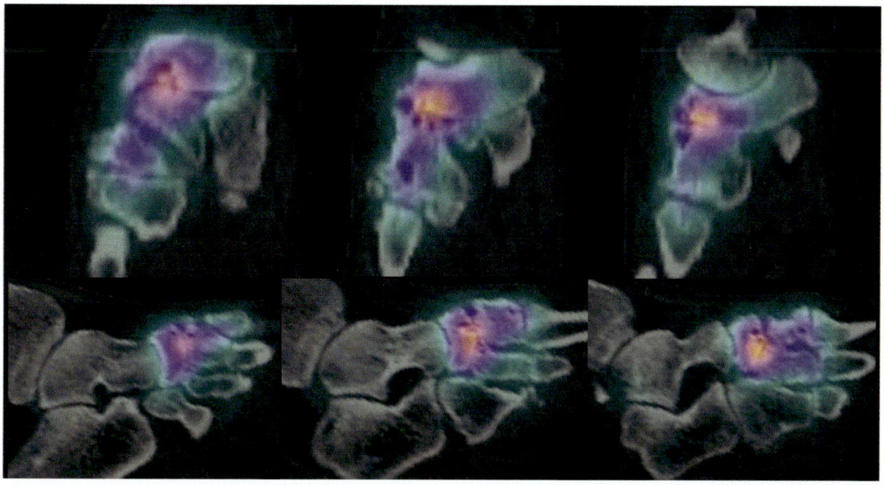

**Fig. 4.15** SPECT-CT of the right foot demonstrates intense isotope uptake at the naviculocuneiform joints with relative quiescence of the talonavicular joint

## 4.8 Critical Appraisal

Maceira and Rochera's classification, based solely on Méary's angle, has been the only one in use for almost two decades since its description in 2004 (Maceira and Rochera 2004). Its end-stage V disease is a reliable endpoint. It is characterized by the talo-cuneiform articulation, whereby the navicular has subluxed medially, the dorsolateral navicular fragment has extruded dorsally and the talar head articulates directly with the lateral cuneiform bones.

Except for Stage I, in which there is no obvious radiological abnormality, the other stages are not as clearly defined. For example, the medial arch should have sagged in 3 feet of Wong-Chung et al. with Maceira Stage V disease (Wong-Chung et al. 2023). Instead, they had notably raised medial arches, which would have been expected in Stage II and not in Stage V disease. Furthermore, the degree of sagging does not correlate with degree of compression. Nor is there correlation between symptomatology and Maceira stages. Therefore, Méary's angle per se does not provide accurate assessment of disease severity. Even Maceira and co-author Monteagudo acknowledged that his classification does not serve as guide to treatment or prognosis (Monteagudo and Maceira 2019). Nevertheless, it describes the pathomechanics well.

In 2004, Maceira and Rochera concluded that all 5 stages of the condition must start in childhood because they had encountered neither a case of compression and fragmentation developing in a normal navicular nor one that had moved on from one stage to the next. They firmly believed in two essential factors for the disease to develop, namely delayed ossification and abnormal compression forces from either an overlong second or a short first metatarsal. They attributed their high '*epidemic*' incidence to the Spanish civil war, which led to famine and caused delayed ossification.

In 2019, they reiterated their previous beliefs and named their first category an 'epidemic' group. However, they also introduced a second category, a '*non*-epidemic' group in which there was no known environmental or nutritional stress that could have caused delayed ossification. This group is said to be made up of child athletes, whose healthy navicular were subjected to '*too much too soon*'. Although they had said in 2004 that they had never seen compression and fragmentation develop in a normal navicular, their third new group, the 'Müller-Weissoid' feet had a previously healthy navicular 'as young adults' and developed disease in late adulthood.

Doyle et al. had found no evidence of past environmental or nutritional stress in their patients (Doyle et al. 2012). Nor do the many recent studies from Egypt (Ahmed et al. 2019) or China (Bai et al. 2023). Even Monteagudo and Maceira (2019) recently remarked that, except for an occasional new attendance from the epidemic group, most of their new cases give no past history of nutritional or environmental stress (Monteagudo and Maceira 2019). This may indicate that perhaps only one factor is essential for development of the disease, namely mechanical causes. However, since not all index minus feet develop Müller-Weiss disease, there must be another as yet unidentified responsible factor.

Wong-Chung et al. identified 23 "Müller-Weissoid' and 3 "reverse Müller-Weissoid" in 95 of their feet. Apart from these, neither their other late-onset nor their early-onset patients had previous radiographs demonstrating normality, except perhaps for one near normal navicular in a 9-year-old child in whom disease progression could be observed over a number of years, as shown in their seventh illustration. Knowing when normality changes to pathology hence proves problematic. Considering that none of the early-onset feet has required surgery yet, it is conceivable that all other groups may have developed disease in childhood when the cartilage has no innervation and symptoms then manifest in adulthood, as suggested by Monteagudo and Maceira. The ideal study is a longitudinal one that includes earliest radiographs showing normal naviculars at the earliest age possible. However, this would not be a realistically achievable goal (See also Sect. 1.8.1).

Monteagudo and Maceira defined Müller-Weissoid changes as having developed in feet with previously normal naviculars, but did not specify the joints where disease occurred. They chose to demonstrate these changes in a bilateral case in their fourth illustration. The case shown actually resembles those depicted in Fig. 4.11, namely of a reverse Müller-Weissoid category of which there were 3 in Wong-Chung et al.'s series with compression and degeneration maximal at the naviculocuneiform rather than at the talonavicular joint. On the other hand, compression and degenerative changes were maximal at the talonavicular joint in the 23 Northern Irish Müller-Weissoid feet.

The Northern Irish study hence comprises 23 Müller-Weissoid feet (24%) involving the talonavicular joint predominantly and 3 reverse Müller-Weissoid feet (3%) affecting the naviculocuneiform joints mostly. Monteagudo and Maceira exemplify with a case of bilateral reverse Müller-Weissoid disease, but again do not disclose how many cases there were. It is not known whether the Spanish series contained any Müller-Weissoid feet as defined by affection mostly of the talonavicular joint. Again, as with the early-onset Group 1 disease (See Sects. 4.6 and 4.6.1), there may be geographical differences in disease pattern, which require further investigations.

## 4.9 Summary of Existing Classifications

According to the World Health Organization (WHO), the three main purposes of classifying disease are to ascertain Cause for future prevention, determine best Treatment and estimate Prognosis. Table 4.1 tabulates the 3 main existing classifications of Müller-Weiss disease, their classifiers, characteristics and contributions to Cause, Treatment and Prognosis.

### *4.9.1 Not Another Classification!*

Another paper due to be published by Wong-Chung et al. in the March/April 2024 issue of the Journal of Foot and Ankle Surgery describes the results of selective arthrodesis in 33 out of 64 feet (Wong-Chung et al. 2023). It was first presented at the Annual Meetings of the British Orthopaedic Foot and Ankle Society (BOFAS) in March 2018, (McKenna et al. 2018) of the Irish Orthopaedic Foot and Ankle Society (IOFAS) in April 2019 and of the American Orthopaedic Foot and Ankle Society (AOFAS) in September 2019 (McKenna et al. 2019). However, it did not get accepted for publication until late 2023. Arthrodesis sites were selected according to joints affected as determined by clinical site of pain and tenderness, radiographic site of arthritis and activity on SPECT-CT. Stages were described according to sites of arthrodesis surgery. Thus, surgical stage 1A involved the talonavicular (TN) joint only; surgical stage 1B, the TN and subtalar joints; surgical stage 2, both TN and naviculocuneiform (NC) joints, necessitating talonaviculocuneiform (TNC) arthrodesis; surgical stage 3, both TN and NC joints with fracture or inadequate bone stock at the lateral navicular, requiring TNC arthrodesis and tricortical iliac crest bone graft (TICBG); and surgical stage 4, talonavicular and associated asymmetric varus ankle osteoarthritis in 3 cases, which underwent pantalar arthrodesis or total ankle arthroplasty.

In the interval between 2018 and 2023, the authors studied an additional 31 feet. A total of 95 feet provided the basis for their final grouping system, which was accepted for publication ahead of the surgical staging system despite completion of the latter 5 years earlier. While the surgical staging system considered only the arthrodesis sites, the grouping system takes into account other parameters such as age, presence of a previous radiologically normal navicular and refines upon the anatomical sites involved. Table 4.2 explains the relationship between the earlier surgical staging system and the later grouping system of Wong-Chung et al. Thus, feet from surgical

**Table 4.1** Classifications of Müller-Weiss disease

| | Maceira and Rochera (2004) | Monteagudo and Maceira (2019) | Wong-Chung et al. (2023) | | | | |
|---|---|---|---|---|---|---|---|
| Classifiers | Méary's angle | Previous radiologically normal navicular | 1. Age<br>2. Previous radiologically normal navicular<br>3. Joints affected<br>4. Méary's angle<br>5. Dorsoplantar talo-first metatarsal angle | | | | |
| Categories | (5 Stages) | (3 Categories) | (3 Groups and 3 Sub-Groups) | | Characteristics | | |
| | Stage I: No bony anomaly on X-Ray | 1. Epidemic | Group 1<br>Early-onset | Youngest | Greatest compression and extrusion | Lowest Kite's | Fracture in 91% |
| | Stage II: Méary's angle apex dorsal | 2. Non-Epidemic | Group 2<br>Late-onset | Müller-Weissoid | Lowest compression and extrusion | Highest Kite's | No fracture |
| | Stage III: Méary's angle neutral | 3. Müller-Weissoid | Group 3A<br>Late-onset | Late-onset TN only | | | No fracture |
| | Stage IV: Méary's angle sags | | Group 3B<br>Late-onset | Late-onset TN > NC | Highest incidence of Maceira Stage V | | Fracture in 65% |
| | Stage V: Talocuneiform articulation | | Group 3C<br>Late-onset | Late-onset NC > TN | Greatest degree of midfoot abduction<br>Greatest overlength of second metatarsal | | Fracture in 32% |
| | (Stage V is a reliable end-point) | | (or Reverse Müller-Weiss disease) | | | | |
| Cause | 1. Delayed ossification of navicular from nutritional deficiency | 1. Delayed ossification of navicular from nutritional deficiency | No nutritional or environmental stress | | | | |

(continued)

**Table 4.1** (continued)

| | Maceira and Rochera (2004) | Monteagudo and Maceira (2019) | Wong-Chung et al. (2023) | |
|---|---|---|---|---|
| | 2. Long second metatarsal or brachymetatarsia of first ray | 2. Long second metatarsal or brachymetatarsia of first ray | Long second metatarsal or brachymetatarsia of first ray | |
| | Describes pathomechanics | 3. Strenuous sports at young age causing "too much stress too soon" | | |
| Treatment | Does not guide treatment | Does not guide treatment | Group 1 Early-onset | No surgery required so far at age of up to 33 years |
| | | | Group 2 M-Woid | Talonavicular / Double Medial / Triple Arthrodesis |
| | | | Group 3A TN only | Talonavicular / Double Medial / Triple Arthrodesis |
| | | | Group 3B TN > NC | Talonaviculocuneiform arthrodesis ± TICBG if fracture or poor bone stock at lateral navicular [a,b] (Consider talonavicular arthrodesis only) |
| | | | Group 3C NC > TN | [c] Talonaviculocuneiform arthrodesis ± TICBG if fracture or poor bone stock at lateral navicular |
| | | | Reverse Müller-Weissoid disease | Talonaviculocuneiform + Tarsometatarsal Arthrodesis |
| Prognosis | No guide to prognosis | No guide to prognosis | To be determined by future studies | |

*Abbreviations* TN, talonavicular joint; NC, naviculocuneiform joint; M-Woid, Müller-Weissoid; Double Medial, arthrodesis of talonavicular and subtalar joints; TICBG, tricortical iliac crest bone graft

[a]Consider reducing medial talonavicular subluxation and perform talonavicular arthrodesis only

[b]Consider talonavicular arthrodesis only if NC joints are asymptomatic

[c]Naviculocuneiform joints need to be included in fusion as they are, by definition, more involved than the talonavicular joint

stages 1A and 1B would come under either Group 2 Müller-Weissoid and Group 3A affecting the talonavicular joint only, and undergo the same types of arthrodesis, namely talonavicular, triple or double medial arthrodesis (solid arrows). Groups 3B and 3C feet affecting both TN and NC joints would have undergone TNC arthrodesis as in surgical stage 2 or TNC arthrodesis with TICBG as in surgical stage 3, in case of fracture or inadequate bone stock at the lateral navicular (compound arrows).

## 4.10 Need for a Common Platform

"A classification allows the world to compare and share data in a consistent and standard way between hospitals, regions and countries, and over periods of time" (WHO).

Müller-Weiss disease remains poorly understood still partly due to overlap with other affections of the navicular, but largely also because of the considerable variation in how the condition is diagnosed and the lack of uniformity in the way it is reported since first described in 1927. For example, as already discussed in Sect. 4.8, Wong-Chung et al. designate Müller-Weissoid as disease occurring in a previously normal navicular predominantly at the talonavicular joint, and reverse Müller-Weissoid as disease developing in a hitherto normal navicular mostly at the naviculocuneiform joint (Wong-Chung et al. 2023). On the other hand, Monteagudo and Maceira exemplify their Müller-Weissoid changes with a case of bilateral reverse Müller-Weissoid disease (Monteagudo and Maceira 2019).

Similarly, the 13 adolescent feet of Ahmed et al. displayed a reverse Müller-Weiss pattern (Ahmed et al. 2019). They had no fracture of the lateral corner and tended to have marked midfoot abduction with less medial talonavicular subluxation, which would explain their rationale for a lateral column lengthening. Wong-Chung et al.'s series comprised 11 young feet which did not exhibit the same pattern, with a tendency to fracture at the lateral corner of the navicular, more marked medial talonavicular subluxation and lesser degrees of midfoot abduction.

Even Maceira acknowledged that his classification does not guide treatment or prognosis, as Méary's angle bears very little correlation with symptomatology. Nonetheless, it remains the only one in wide usage, its proposed modification by Mayich not having gained much recognition. As a result, most studies group all their cases together, regardless of which perinavicular joints are affected and to what extent. This may explain why the literature reflects a distinct lack of gold standard in the surgical treatment of Müller-Weiss disease, for want of a more comprehensive classification.

Lu et al. attempted to make recommendations based upon Maceira gradings (Lu et al. 2014). They advocated core decompression or excision of the lateral navicular fragment for symptomatic Maceira Stage I or II. For Stages III and IV, they believed isolated talonavicular arthrodesis to be adequate. For Stage V, they advocated triple, double or talonaviculocuneiform arthrodesis with abundant bone graft. Some centers universally perform isolated talonavicular arthrodesis utilizing either a lateral tension

**Table 4.2** Relationship between the surgical stages and grouping system of Müller-Weiss disease

**Table 4.2** Relationship between the Surgical Stages and Grouping System of Müller-Weiss Disease

| Wong-Chung et al., 2024 Surgical stages | | | Wong-Chung et al., 2023 Grouping system | |
|---|---|---|---|---|
| Sites of arthritis | Surgery performed | Stage | | |
| Talonavicular arthritis | Talonavicular arthrodesis | Stage 1A | Group 2 Late-onset Müller-Weissoid | Talonavicular Double Medial or Triple Arthrodesis |
| Talonavicular + Subtalar arthritis | Triple arthrodesis or double medial arthrodesis | Stage 1B | Group 3A Late-onset TN only | Talonavicular Double Medial or Triple Arthrodesis |
| Talonavicular + Naviculocuneiform | Talonaviculocuneiform arthrodesis | Stage 2 | Group 3B Late-onset TN > NC | Talonaviculocuneiform arthrodesis<br>± TICBG if fracture or inadequate bone stock at lateral navicular<br>[a,b] (Consider talonavicular arthrodesis only) |
| Talonavicular + Naviculocuneiform with fracture or inadequate bone stock at lateral navicular | Talonaviculocuneiform arthrodesis with TICBG | Stage 3 | Group 3C Late-onset NC > TN | [c] Talonaviculocuneiform arthrodesis<br>± TICBG if fracture or inadequate bone stock at lateral navicular |
| | | | Reverse Müller-Weissoid disease | Talonaviculocuneiform + Tarsometatarsal Arthrodesis |
| Talonavicular + Asymmetric varus ankle arthritis | Pantalar arthrodesis or Total ankle arthroplasty | Stage 4 | | |

*Abbreviations:* Double Medial, arthrodesis of talonavicular and subtalar joints; TN, talonavicular joint; NC, naviculocuneiform joint; TICBG, tricortical iliac crest bone graft.

[a] Consider reducing medial talonavicular subluxation and perform talonavicular arthrodesis only

[b] Consider talonavicular arthrodesis only if NC joints are asymptomatic

[c] Naviculocuneiform joints need to be included in fusion as they are, by definition, more involved than the talonavicular joint.

band principle (Fornaciari et al. 2014) or derotating the talus using a pin distractor to reduce the medial talonavicular subluxationYuan et al. 2019) while others endorse talonaviculocuneiform arthrodesis for all cases with or without an interpositional tricortical iliac crest bone graft (Fernández de Retana et al. 2004; Ahmad 2015; Cao et al. 2012; Yu et al. 2012). Contrary to these empirical approaches, recent authors stress the need to tailor surgery according to the joints involved, the extent of navicular compression, the amount of remaining cancellous bone in the lateral third of the navicular, and the presence of a fracture with detachment and dorsal extrusion of the avascular lateral navicular fragment (Mayich 2016; Cao and Miao 2018; Liu et al. 2022).

Wong-Chung et al. drew an analogy of the current situation to when Marvin Tile put forward his classification of pelvic and acetabular fractures, emphasizing the need to compare like-for-like cases and avoid comparing apples and oranges (Tile 1988, 1995). Similarly, in order to define gold standards of treatment, be it surgical or nonoperative, the authors therefore called for a more standardized fashion of describing Müller-Weiss disease. They propose a combination of Maceira's classification, which is based solely on Méary's angle, and their grouping system, which takes into account (a) age (b) evidence of a previous radiologically normal navicular bone (c) the joints affected (d) dorsoplantar and (e) lateral Méary's angles.

For example, a Wong Group 3A Maceira Stage III will indicate involvement of talonavicular joint only with a neutral Méary's angle. A common adult-onset presentation is of a Wong Group 3B Maceira Stage V, which designates a foot involving the talonavicular more than the naviculocuneiform, with the talar head articulating directly with the lateral cuneiform. Surgery advocated for the Wong Group 3B Maceira Stage V varies widely from (a) in-situ talonavicular arthrodesism, (Lu et al. 2014) to (b) isolated talonavicular arthrodesis using a pin distractor to reduce medial talonavicular subluxation, (Yuan et al. 2019) (c) TNC arthrodesis with TICBG (Mayich 2016; Bai et al. 2023) and (d) a hybrid 4-joint arthrodesis consisting of a triple arthrodesis plus a TICBG between the talar head and lateral cuneiform, leaving NC1 and NC2 untouched (Zhang et al. 2017). And all with reportedly good results!

Using the two descriptions/classifications in conjunction will help determine (a) which groups are more likely to succeed or fail with nonoperative treatment and (b) evaluate results of different surgical modalities such as lateral displacement calcaneal osteotomy or universal use of isolated talonavicular arthrodesis as advocated by Yuan et al. even in cases with marked medial displacement, severe compression and fragmentation of the lateral navicular (Yuan et al. 2019).

**Concluding Remarks**

Maceira's classification, the only one in use for the past twenty years, relies solely on Méary's angle. Even its proponents accept it does not guide treatment or prognosis. Despite these shortcomings, it explains pathomechanics well and its Stage V is a consistent endpoint marked by formation of the talocuneiform articulation.

The grouping system proposed by Wong-Chung et al. in 2023 takes into account age of disease onset, previous evidence of a radiologically normal navicular, the peri-navicular joints affected, dorsoplantar and lateral talo-first metatarsal angles. Of note, its Group 3C describes a previously unrecognized disease pattern with compression more marked at the naviculocuneiform than the talonavicular side. Termed reverse Müller-Weiss disease, it has the greatest second metatarsal overlength and the highest degree of midfoot abduction.

It also exposes geographical variations in pattern of the disease such as dissimilarities between early-onset disease in Egypt and Northern Ireland, and differences between Müller-Weissoid and reverse Müller-Weissoid patterns in Spain and Northern Ireland. There hence exists a real need for a globally encompassing classification for reporting outcomes of operative and nonoperative treatment of Müller-Weiss disease. Only then can gold standards be defined.

A combination of Maceira's stages and Wong groups may provide a more comprehensive way for reporting the disease and outcomes of treatment. The future lies in testing and fine-tuning the proposed combined classification of Maceira and Wong-Chung et al.

## References

Ahmad J. Perinavicular arthrodesis as treatment of advanced navicular osteonecrosis. Tech Foot Ankle Surg. 2015;14:79–87. https://doi.org/10.1097/BTF.0000000000000090.

Ahmed AA, Kandil MI, Tabl EA. Preliminary outcomes of calcaneal lengthening in adolescent flatfoot in Müller-Weiss disease. Foot Ankle Int. 2019;40(7):803–7. https://doi.org/10.1177/1071100719833928.

Bai W, Li Y, Shen G, Zhang H, Li X, Zhu Y. Talonavicular-cuneiform arthrodesis for the treatment of Müller-Weiss: mid-term results of 15 cases after 5 years. BMC Musculoskelet Disord. 2023;24(1):178. https://doi.org/10.1186/s12891-023-06293-1.

Cao HH, Tang KL, Xu JZ. Peri-navicular arthrodesis for the stage III Müller-Weiss disease. Foot Ankle Int. 2012;33(6):475–8. https://doi.org/10.3113/FAI.2012.0475.

Cao L, Miao XD. Selective arthrodesis for treatment of symptomatic Müller-Weiss disease. Foot and Ankle Orthopaedics. 2018;3:3. https://doi.org/10.1177/2473011418S00033.

Doyle T, Napier RJ, Wong-Chung J. Recognition and management of Müller-Weiss disease. Foot Ankle Int. 2012;33(4):275–81. https://doi.org/10.3113/FAI.2012.0275.

Fernández de Retana P, Maceira E, Fernández-Valencia JA, Suso S. Arthrodesis of the talonavicular-cuneiform joints in Müller-Weiss disease. Foot Ankle Clin. 2004;9(1):65–72. https://doi.org/10.1016/s1083-7515(03)00175-x

Fornaciari P, Gilgen A, Zwicky L, Lang TH, Hintermann B. Isolated talonavicular fusion with tension band for Müller-Weiss syndrome. Foot Ankle Int. 2014;35(12):1316–22. https://doi.org/10.1177/1071100714548197.

Kellgren JH, Lawrence JS. Radiological assessment of osteo-arthrosis. Annals Rheumatic Diseases. 1957;16:494–502.

Lu CK, Fu YC, Cheng YM, Huang PJ. Isolated talonavicular arthrodesis for Müller-Weiss disease. Kaohsiung J Med Sci. 2014;30:471–6. https://doi.org/10.1016/j.kjms.2014.05.001.

Liu W, Chen Y, Zeng G, Yang T, Ma M, Song W. Individual surgical treatment of stage IV Müller-Weiss disease according to CT/MRI examination: a retrospective study of 12 cases. Front Surg. 2022;17(9): 694597. https://doi.org/10.3389/fsurg.2022.694597.

Maceira E, Rochera R. Müller-Weiss disease: clinical and biomechanical features. Foot Ankle Clin. 2004;9(1):105–25. https://doi.org/10.1016/S1083-7515(03)00153-0.

Monteagudo M, Maceira E. Management of Müller-Weiss disease. Foot Ankle Clin. 2019;24(1):89–105. https://doi.org/10.1016/j.fcl.2018.09.006.

Mayich, DJ. The treatment of Mueller-Weiss disease: a systematic approach. Tech Foot Ankle Surg. 2016;15(2):59–73. https://doi.org/10.1097/BTF.0000000000000088

McKenna R, Wong J, Tucker A. Muller-Weiss disease; proposed classification and treatment algorithm. BOFAS 2018;Podium Abstract.

McKenna R, Wong-Chung J, Tucker A. Müller Weiss disease: radiological evaluation and proposed treatment algorithm. Foot Ankle Orthop. 2019;4(4). https://doi.org/10.1177/2473011419S00055

Tile M. Pelvic fractures—should they be fixed. J Bone Joint Surg. 1988;70B:1–12. https://doi.org/10.1302/0301-620X.70B1.3276697.

Tile M. Fractures of the pelvis and acetabulum. 2nd ed. Baltimore, MD: Williams & Wilkins; 1995. p. 3.

Wong-Chung J, Blythe A, Lynch-Wong M, McKenna R, Wilson A, Stephens M. Outcomes of selective arthrodesis based on joints affected in 33 Feet with Müller-Weiss disease. J Foot Ankle Surg. 2024;63(2):199–206. https://doi.org/10.1053/j.jfas.2023.11.001

Wong-Chung J, Walls A, Lynch-Wong M, Cassidy R, McKenna R, Wilson A, Stephens M. Towards understanding Müller-Weiss disease from an analysis of 95 cases. Foot Ankle Surg. 2023;29(5):401–11. https://doi.org/10.1016/j.fas.2023.05.004.

Yuan C, Wang C, Zhang C, Huang J, Wang X, Ma X. Derotation of the talus and arthrodesis treatment of stages II-V Müller-Weiss disease: midterm results of 36 cases. Foot Ankle Int. 2019;40(5):506–14. https://doi.org/10.1177/1071100719829457.

Yu G, Zhao Y, Zhou J, Zhang M. Fusion of talonavicular and naviculocuneiform joints for the treatment of Müller-Weiss disease. J Foot Ankle Surg. 2012;51(4):415–9. https://doi.org/10.1053/j.jfas.2012.04.004.

Zhang H, Li J, Qiao Y, Yu J, Cheng Y, Liu Y, Gao C, Li J. Open triple fusion versus TNC arthrodesis in the treatment of Mueller-Weiss disease. J Orthop Surg Res. 2017;12:13. https://doi.org/10.1186/s13018-017-0513-3.

# Chapter 5
# Nonoperative Treatment of Müller-Weiss Disease

**Abstract** All feet with Müller-Weiss disease should undergo an adequate trial of nonoperative treatment. The degree of midfoot abduction may determine success or failure of nonoperative treatment. Patients with heel varus and flatfeet may benefit from a lateral heel wedge combined with a medial arch support. It would be more useful to study which Wong groups will benefit from nonoperative treatment.

**Keywords** Müller-Weiss disease · Nonoperative treatment · Orthotics · Lateral heel wedge · Pedobarography · Midfoot abduction

### Introduction

All feet should undergo a trial of nonoperative treatment for a minimum period of 3 months. This consists of rest, activity modification, weight reduction, non-steroidal anti-inflammatory agents, stretching exercises, shoe modification with rocker-bottom soles and custom-made orthoses to offload the affected joints (Ruiz-Escobar et al. 2020 ). Rocker-bottom shoes may alleviate perinavicular pain. They limit midfoot motion and improve the transition from the first to the third rocker. Monteagudo and Maceira (Spain, 2019) claims good pain relief from magnetotherapy in half of their cases (Monteagudo and Maceira 2019).

This Chapter also analyzes possible predictors for failure of nonoperative treatment.

## 5.1 Lateral Heel Wedge with Medial Arch Support

Based on comparative pedobarographic studies, Hetsroni et al. (Israel, 2007) recommended use of a rigid orthotic support with the heel posted in valgus (Hetsroni et al. 2007). Compared to 18 normal feet, 8 feet with Müller-Weiss disease had shown significantly higher pressures in the midfoot ($p < 0.05$) and lower plantar pressures along the medial part of the heel ($p = 0.015$) and toe segments ($p < 0.01$).

© The Author(s), under exclusive license to Springer Nature Switzerland AG 2024 
J. Wong-Chung, *Comprehensive Guide to Müller-Weiss Disease*,
https://doi.org/10.1007/978-3-031-66644-5_5

Monteagudo and Maceira had noticed that patients with Müller-Weiss disease, when referred to the orthotist, were being fitted with a medial arch support and a medial heel wedge (Monteagudo and Maceira 2019). Patients were not satisfied and complained of lateral ankle instability and peroneal pain. When the authors realized that heel varus was a constant feature of the condition, the orthotics were altered to a medial arch support to counteract navicular sag and a 10- to 12-mm lateral heel wedge to control subtalar supination. The new design of orthotics proved more effective and avoided the need for surgery in 80% of cases, regardless of disease stages.

Li et al. (2017) stated that a positive response from such an orthotic also constituted a good indication for a lateral displacement calcaneal osteotomy (Li et al. 2017).

The corollary should be that patients who do not respond favourably to orthotics may be expected not to respond well to surgery. However, Monteagudo and Maceira (2019) subsequently reported no correlation between a favourable or unfavourable response to orthotics and good outcome from surgery (Monteagudo and Maceira (2019). In fact, patients who showed no improvement with orthotics, also experienced considerable improvement following surgery. Therefore, failure to get better with orthotics constitutes yet another indication for calcaneal osteotomy. This last statement seems at odds with their previous 2017 criterion of a positive response to orthotics as a prerequisite for lateral displacement calcaneal osteotomy (Li et al. (2017).

It should be noted that Wong-Chung et al. reported that only 33% of feet with Müller-Weiss disease had a combination of heel varus and flatfoot (Wong-Chung et al. 2023). This means that not all feet would benefit from a lateral heel wedge with medial arch support.

## 5.2 Factors Determining Failure of Nonoperative Treatment

Harnroongoj et al. (Thailand, 2021) actively sought out demographic and radiographic differences that would determine success or failure of nonoperative treatment (Harnroongroj et al.2021). They retrospectively reviewed 68 patients with Müller-Weiss disease, 39 of whom responded successfully to conservative treatment. The remaining 29 failed to respond to conservative measures and proceeded to surgery. All patients underwent the same conservative treatment protocol, which consisted of short courses of non-steroidal anti-inflammatory drugs and an offloading full-length semirigid insole with medial longitudinal arch support for a minimum period of 3 months.

For each patient, they documented demographic data such as age and gender, BMI, smoking habit, duration of nonoperative treatment, Visual Analog Scale (VAS) for pain and walking disability, Foot and Ankle Outcome Score (FAOS) for pain, symptoms and activities of daily living, and quality of life subscales. Radiographic assessment included measurement of calcaneal pitch, lateral Méary's and dorsoplantar talo-first metatarsal (DPTFM) or dorsoplantar Méary's angles. Arthritis at the talonavicular and naviculocuneiform joints were graded according to the degree of joint space narrowing and amount of osteophyte formation on both dorsoplantar and lateral radiographs, as described by Menz et al. (2019). Logistic regression analysis was utilized to identify descriptive factors for failure of nonoperative treatment.

The group treated conservatively with 'success' was significantly older (63.2 $\pm$ 8.34 years) compared to the 'failure' group (56.8 $\pm$ 9.77 years) ($p = 0.005$). However, multivariate analysis did not demonstrate age as a statistically significant descriptive factor for failure of conservative treatment. No significant differences existed between the two groups with regards to gender, BMI, heavy smoking, duration of symptoms and Maceira staging.

With respect to clinical outcomes, the group in which conservative treatment failed had more severe VAS scores for pain and walking disability, and also worse FAOS scores for pain, activities of daily living and quality of life subscales ($p < 0.05$) than the successful group. In other words, symptoms in the feet that did not respond to nonoperative measures and proceeded to surgery were much more severe.

As regards radiographic parameters, the successful group had (a) significantly lower calcaneal pitch angle (8.21 $\pm$ 5.94°) compared to the failure group (11.3 $\pm$ 6.12°) ($p = 0.041$), (b) less midfoot abduction as measured by the DPTFM or dorsoplantar Méary's angle (4.0 $\pm$ 10°) compared to the failure group (13 $\pm$ 18°) ($p = 0.001$), (c) significantly lower presence of talonavicular arthritis (41%) compared to the failure group (79.3%) ($p = 0.002$) and (d) lower severity score for radiographic talonavicular osteoarthritis of 1 $\pm$ 2 compared to 4 $\pm$ 2 in the failure group ($p < 0.001$).

By univariate analysis, statistically significant differences existed between the 2 groups for age, calcaneal pitch angle, AP Méary's angle, radiographic talonavicular and naviculocuneiform arthritis ($p < 0.2$). However, multivariate analysis demonstrated only 2 significant negative prognostic indicators for failure of nonoperative treatment: (a) presence of radiographic talonavicular osteoarthritis ($p = 0.004$) and (b) midfoot abduction with a dorsoplantar Méary's angle of greater than 13 degrees ($p < 0.001$). The authors inferentially chose 13° as the amount of midfoot abduction that would lead to failure of nonoperative treatment, because it was the median value in the failure group.

Interestingly, Harnroongoj et al. concluded with the recommendation that any new classification should take into account the degree of radiological talonavicular arthritis and amount of midfoot abduction. Unaware of this last statement, Wong-Chung et al. (2023, Northern Ireland) did take into consideration the dorsoplantar talo-first metatarsal angle in their grouping system (Wong-Chung et al. 2021). In their series of 95 feet, they found that the late-onset Group 3C reverse Müller-Weiss disease had the highest degree of midfoot abduction ($p < 0.002$) (See Chap. 4 on Classification Systems). There was also a strong correlation between DPTFM and lateral Méary's angles ($p < 0.001$).

Of the 95 feet with Müller-Weiss disease, 37 (39%) proceeded to surgery after failed nonoperative treatment. The remaining 58 feet either responded to conservative treatment or were not symptomatic enough to warrant surgery. Our unpublished data shows no significant difference between average DPTFM angles in operated (−6.4°) and non-operated (−5.3°) feet ($p = 0.928$) (Table 5.1). Negative values refer to midfoot abduction whereas positive values refer to midfoot adduction. The DPTFM angle exceeded −13° (range, −15 to −37°) in just 8 of the 37 feet (21.6%) that proceeded to surgery.

## 5.3 Surgical Conversion Rate

At 5-years' follow-up, Harnroongroj and Chuckpaiwong et al. (Thailand, 2021) described a 56.3% failure of nonoperative treatment in 32 patients (Harnroongroj et al.2018). From the same institution earlier, Nepal and Chuckpaiwong (Thailand, 2019) had reported successful outcome in a 61-year-old woman with Group 3B Stage V disease treated by orthotics alone for 9 years (Nepal and Chuckpaiwong 2019). In 95 feet, Wong-Chung et al. recorded a lower surgical conversion rate of 39% (Wong-Chung et al. 2023).

## 5.4 Recommended Follow-Up Régime for Nonoperative Treatment

For monitoring of nonoperative treatment, Angthong et al. (Thailand, 2023) recommended regular follow-up at 6 weeks, 3 months, 6 months and annually thereafter (Angthong et al.2023).

**Concluding Remarks**

Initial management of Müller-Weiss disease is always an adequate trial of nonoperative treatment. Various centers have advocated use of a lateral heel wedge combined with a medial arch support, based on the concept of paradoxical pes planus varus and obligatory heel varus as hallmark deformities of the condition. This approach is only appropriate when true heel varus exists, since only 33% of cases were found to have heel varus in a major study using hindfoot alignment radiographs.

Conversion rate to surgery varies between 39 to 56%. Besides the presence of talonavicular arthritis, it has been postulated that midfoot abduction with a dorsoplantar talo-first metatarsal (DPTFM) angle of greater than 13° would signify a greater likelihood of need for surgery. However, the Author's own experience with 37 operated feet does not corroborate this, the DPTFM angle exceeding 13° in only 21% of feet that proceeded to surgery.

None of the Group 1 early-onset disease has required surgery so far. It may be more useful to correlate outcomes of nonoperative treatment with the Wong groups and presence or absence of heel varus instead.

**Table 5.1** The dorsoplantar Talo-first metatarsal angle in Müller-Weiss disease

| | | Operated (37) | | | | | Nonoperated (58) | | | | |
|---|---|---|---|---|---|---|---|---|---|---|---|
| | | Number of Feet | Range | | Average | Mean | Number of Feet | Range | | Average | Mean |
| Group 1 | Early-onset | 0 | | | | | 11 | 9 | −5.9 | 1.93 | 1.7 |
| Group 2 | Müller-Weissoid | 8 | 7.2 | −7 | −0.23 | 1 | 15 | 13 | −2.1 | −3.2 | −1.5 |
| Group 3A | Talonavicular only | 11 | 7.2 | −24 | −6.8 | −8 | 5 | 12 | −13 | −2.6 | −3 |
| Group 3B | Talonavicular > naviculocuneiform | 12 | 4 | −18 | −4.75 | −4 | 8 | 4.9 | −11 | −5.3 | −8 |
| Group 3C | Naviculocuneiform > talonavicular (Reverse Müller-Weiss disease) | 6 | −4 | −37 | −17.33 | −12 | 19 | 2 | −23 | −11.9 | −11 |

Negative values denote midfoot abduction
Positive values denote midfoot adduction

## References

Angthong C, Younger ASE, Chuckpaiwong B, Harnroongroj T, Veljkovic A. A novel update on the management of Müller-Weiss disease: presentation of a treatment algorithm. Cartilage. 2023;18:19476035231205684. https://doi.org/10.1177/19476035231205684.

Harnroongroj T, Tharmviboonsri T, Chuckpaiwong B. Müller-Weiss disease: the descriptive factors of failure conservative treatment. Foot Ankle Int. 2021;42(8):1022–30. https://doi.org/10.1177/10711007211002826.

Harnroongroj T, Chuckpaiwong B. Muller-Weiss disease. The survivorship of conservative treatment to 5-year follow-up. Foot and Ankle Orthop. 2018;3(3). https://doi.org/10.1177/2473011418S00241

Hetsroni I, Nyska M, Ayalon M. Plantar pressure distribution in patients with Müller-Weiss disease. Foot Ankle Int. 2007;28(2):237–41. https://doi.org/10.3113/FAI.2007.0237.

Li S-Y, Myerson MS, Monteagudo M, Maceira E. Efficacy of calcaneus osteotomy for treatment of symptomatic Müller-Weiss disease. Foot Ankle Int. 2017;38(3):261–9. https://doi.org/10.1177/1071100716677741.

Menz HB, Munteanu SE, Landorf KB, Zammit GV, Cicuttini FM. Radiographic evaluation of foot osteoarthritis: sensitivity of radiographic variables and relationship to symptoms. Osteoarthritis Cartilage. 2009;17(3):298–303. https://doi.org/10.1016/j.joca.2008.07.011.

Monteagudo M, Maceira E. Management of Müller-Weiss disease. Foot Ankle Clin. 2019;24:89–105. https://doi.org/10.1016/j.fcl.2018.09.006.

Nepal S, Chuckpaiwong B. Müller-Weiss Disease. J Med Imaging Case Rep. 2019;3(1):14–15. https://doi.org/10.17756/micr.2019-025

Ruiz-Escobar J, Viladot-Pericé R, Álvarez-Goenaga F, Ruiz-Escobar P, Rodríguez-Boronat E. Tratamiento con soportes plantares en la enfermedad de Müller-Weiss. Reporte preliminar [Treatment with plantar supports in Müller-Weiss disease. Preliminary report]. Acta Ortop Mex. 2020;34(2):112–118.

Wong-Chung J, Walls A, Lynch-Wong M, Cassidy R, McKenna R, Wilson A, Stephens M. Towards understanding Müller-Weiss disease from an analysis of 95 cases. Foot Ankle Surg. 2023;29(5):401–11. https://doi.org/10.1016/j.fas.2023.05.004.

Wong-Chung J, McKenna R, Tucker A, Gibson D, Datta P. Radiographic analysis of Muller-Weiss disease. Foot Ankle Surg. 2021;27(5):501–509. https://doi.org/10.1016/j.fas.2020.06.009

# Chapter 6
# Planning for Surgery in Müller-Weiss Disease

**Abstract** As with any surgery, especially major, preoperative planning plays a very important role in success of the surgical procedure. Carefully select the joints to be fused by clinical assessment of pain and tenderness at the various perinavicular joints, confirming with diagnostic injections as necessary. Review the radiographs and SPECT-CT to determine amount of necrotic bone and remaining bone stock. All required instrumentation and implants should be available in the operating room, including allograft bone and other biologics. This author prefers autologous tricortical iliac crest bone graft to replace large bony defects. Aim to reduce any medial talonavicular subluxation. Reduction of the navicular from its displaced plantar and medial location to the apex of the medial arch will automatically restore medial column length, correct the medial arch and midfoot abduction. Good joint preparation and stable fixation will ensure a favourable milieu for union.

**Keywords** Müller-Weiss disease · Surgical planning · SPECT-CT · Joint selection · Patient optimization · Bone graft

## Introduction

As for any surgical procedure, however minor or major, preoperative planning is essential. Since surgery of Müller-Weiss disease consists mostly of arthrodesis ± calcaneal osteotomy, joints to be fused require careful selection through physical examination, plain radiography, SPECT-CT ± MRI. Informed consent including knowing what to expect in the postoperative period undoubtedly improve the patient's surgical journey.

© The Author(s), under exclusive license to Springer Nature Switzerland AG 2024

J. Wong-Chung, *Comprehensive Guide to Müller-Weiss Disease*,
https://doi.org/10.1007/978-3-031-66644-5_6

## 6.1 Aims of Surgery

The goals of surgical intervention are (1) pain relief by arthrodesis of symptomatic arthritic joints and (2) realignment including restoration of the medial longitudinal arch to produce a stable, balanced, plantigrade foot (Mohiuddin et al. 2014). Some surgeons perform lateral displacement calcaneal osteotomy only without arthrodesis (Li et al. 2017; Monteagudo and Maceira 2019).

## 6.2 Indications

Failure of at least 3 months of nonoperative treatment.

## 6.3 Principles of Arthrodesis Surgery

The following principles will guide the preoperative evaluation and planning (Mayich 2016; Ahmed et al. 2019).

1. First, determine which joints are arthritic and symptomatic enough to require fusion by way of clinical examination, SPECT-CT and diagnostic injections.
2. Provision of a biological milieu favorable for healing.
    a. Thorough joint preparation for optimal healing.
    b. Removal of all non-viable bone that have no ability to heal.
3. Determine amount of bone loss and bone stock available for fixation.
4. Determine degree of medial column shortening.
5. Consider need for bone graft and/or bone graft substitutes.
    a. Autograft v/s allograft.
    b. Structural v/s morselized graft.
6. Provision of stability until arthrodesis unites.
7. Ensure availability of required surgical devices and implants in the operating room.

Mayich considered it important to use orthopaedic principles while also remaining flexible, because "of considerable variability in anatomy and characteristics of the disease making no single strategy likely to be the correct method" (Mayich 2016).

## 6.4 Preoperative Evaluation and Planning

Careful preoperative workup enables selection and planning of appropriate surgical procedure. It can be performed at a Preoperative Assessment (POA) or Consent Clinic.

(a) In selecting which joints to fuse, perform a careful physical examination of the foot. In particular, examine for localized tenderness at the talonavicular, subtalar, calcaneocuboid and naviculocuneiform joints.
(b) Assess heel position by inspection and palpation. With the patient standing with both feet at shoulder width, the medial border of both feet parallel and the toes pointing directly forwards at the examiner, determine the presence of a positive peekaboo sign as described by Beals and Manoli (Beals and Manoli 1996). The examiner should view the feet at ankle level and not from above at knee level. Another good way to assess heel orientation is when the patient is lying supine. The examiner holds the heel in the palm of the hand and gently moves the heel towards maximum eversion. A combination of tactile feedback and position sense gives a more accurate assessment of spatial orientation of the heel.
(c) Appropriate hindfoot and forefoot weight-bearing radiographs are analyzed as described in Chap. 3 on Radiographic Features. The hindfoot alignment view is useful as a cross-check against clinical heel position.
(d) SPECT-CT has proven valuable in determining which perinavicular joints are metabolically active. Interpreted in conjunction with site of clinical tenderness, it will assist the physician in selection of joint arthrodesis (Sun et al. 2022). This usually consists of isolated talonavicular, double medial, triple or talonaviculo-cuneiform arthrodesis ± lateral displacement calcaneal osteotomy or subtalar arthrodesis.
(e) In the presence of tenderness and increased isotope uptake at the subtalar joint, heel varus can be simultaneously corrected by combining a lateral closing wedge subtalar arthrodesis with talonavicular or talonaviculocuneiform fusion.
(f) Alternatively, one may select isolated lateral displacement calcaneal osteotomy as advocated by Li et al. to correct heel varus if present (Li et al. 2017). The patient should however be forewarned that pain may persist and arthrodesis may then be required.

## 6.5 Optimizing the Patient Before Surgery

Ensure patient is not or has stopped smoking and/or vaping for at least 6 weeks prior to surgery. Non-steroidal anti-inflammatory drugs (NSAID) should be discontinued for 10 to 14 days prior to surgery. Since most of the Müller-Weiss patients are female, oral contraceptive or hormone replacement therapy should be withheld for 6 weeks before surgery. Not infrequently, patients wrongly assume they can resume smoking, NSAID's or hormone therapy once the surgery has happened, placing them at higher risk of nonunion and thromboembolic phenomena.

Informed consent is obtained for arthrodesis ± calcaneal osteotomy ± harvesting of autologous calcaneal or iliac crest bone graft where anticipated. Risks of bleeding, infection, wound problems, thromboembolism, nonunion, load transfer and need for future procedure are explained. Inform patient of postoperative immobilization protocol in cast followed by walker boot.

## 6.6 Readying the Operating Room

It is important to have all the necessary equipment and biologics in the operating room prior to start.

Graft material and biologics: Femoral head allograft. This author prefers autograft to allograft. BMAC (Bone Marrow Aspirate Concentrate) kit.

Implants as have been used by the Author:

I. Isolated talonavicular arthrodesis:

- Compression staples e.g. Uni-CP (Integra LifeSciences Corp, Plainsboro, NJ)
- 4.5 mm cannulated Low Profile Screw (Arthrex Inc, Naples, FL)
- Midfoot CP plate (Stryker GmbH, Selzach, Switzerland)

II. Double medial arthrodesis

- As per talonavicular arthrodesis plus
- 6.7 mm cannulated Low Profile screw (Arthrex Inc, Naples, FL) – for the subtalar component in antegrade or retrograde mode

III. Triple arthrodesis – as per talonavicular and subtalar joints.

IV. Talonaviculocuneiform arthrodesis ± interpositional tricortical iliac crest bone graft

- Medial column fixation with Proximal Arch Plate (Paragon 28, Englewood, CO)
- Dorsal locking $2^8$ plates (Paragon 28, Englewood, CO)
- Caspar compression and distraction device (Paragon 28, Englewood, CO). It has a compression mode to assist reduction and a distraction mode to assist joint preparation.

## 6.7 Patient Positioning and Surgical Preparation

Supine position. Floppy semi-lateral position or bump beneath the ipsilateral buttock if subtalar arthrodesis or calcaneal osteotomy is also envisaged.

Prep the iliac crest especially if harvest of a tricortical iliac crest bone graft is anticipated.

## 6.8 Operative Considerations

1. Exposure
2. Joint preparation
3. Intraoperative determination of medial column reduction
4. Graft material ± biological augmentation
5. Fixation strategies

### 6.8.1 *Exposure*

- Similar to dual approaches for fracture of the talar neck, medial only or dorsal only approach is not adequate.
- Medial incision between tibialis anterior and tibialis posterior.
- In the dorsal approach, tibialis anterior tendon can be retracted to either side.

### 6.8.2 *Joint Preparation*

- All necrotic bone must be removed.
- Should the avascular lateral navicular fragment be morselized for bone graft? Probably not. Dead bone does not heal and leads to nonunion (Wong-Chung et al. 2023).
- Prepare talus, remaining navicular and cuneiform bones with high-speed burr and saline irrigation. Some surgeons would avoid powered instruments and prefer manual preparation using flexible chisel and curette.
- Let down tourniquet to ensure there is a healthy bleeding bony bed.

### 6.8.3 *Medial Column Reduction*

Mayich utilizes feducial markers or 30-mm calibration balls in preoperative imaging for accurate measurement of length of the medial column (Mayich 2016). Four measurements are made on dorsoplantar standing radiographs and CT scan of both feet to allow comparison.

I. Amount of remaining viable medial navicular bone.
II. Distance between talar head and distal border of medial cuneiform gives an indication of the amount of bone loss and/or degree of medial subluxation of

the navicular tuberosity and hence the measurement required to restore medial column length.

III. Distance between talar head and the medial and lateral edges of the distal border of intermediate cuneiform for a more global assessment of medial column loss. It provides useful backup measurements intraoperatively for confirmation of reduction.

IV. Distance between talar head and proximal border of lateral cuneiform. Although very difficult to measure intraoperatively, it gives a 'ballpark' estimate of graft size.

On lateral standing radiographs, amount of bone loss is estimated by comparing lengths of the talocuneiform lines. Amount of talar neck available for proximal fixation can also be readily measured.

Mayich acknowledges the considerable inter and intraobserver errors when performing and applying these measurements, which may not be as helpful in bilateral disease. He preps both feet to allow clinical assessment of realignment. He places a laminar spreader in the defect at the midfoot. It is distracted according to the preoperative measurements and until hindfoot alignment of both feet match. Provisional fixation is obtained with K-wires and reduction confirmed by intraoperative hindfoot alignment views.

Mayich goes to great lengths to estimate loss of length of the medial column and required size of interpositional graft. Bai et al. simplify this process (Bai et al. 2023). They reason that shortening of the medial column is due to internal rotation of the navicular and medial subluxation at the talonavicular joint. The anteroposterior dimension of the medial third of the navicular itself remains otherwise largely unaffected, as compression and fragmentation occurs mainly at the lateral one to two thirds. By (a) releasing the plantar ligament and plantar soft tissue attachments of the navicular leaving only the insertion of the posterior tibial tendon medially and (b) excising osteophytes laterally at the 4-corners as defined by Doyle et al. (Doyle et al. 2012) they are able to push and reduce the medial navicular remnant laterally and upwards to its correct position at the apex of the medial arch. This step alone restores medial arch height and medial column length. The lateral defect can then be measured and a tricortical iliac crest fashioned for interference fit. (See also Chapter on Talonaviculocuneiform arthrodesis).

### *6.8.4 Graft*

Bony defects commonly range from 3 to 5 cm in size. The graft employed must contribute to structural stability as well as satisfy the biological requirements for healing. A good interference fit is critical for biomechanical stability and a stable construct.

- Autograft. The tricortical iliac crest bone graft (TICBG) remains the gold standard.
- Allograft with or without synthetic growth factors and BMAC augmentation
- Synthetic bone graft

### 6.8.5 *Fixation Using Combined Compressive and Spanning Methods*

Section 6.6 lists the implants used for internal fixation when performing different types of arthrodesis. This section deals with talonaviculocuneiform arthrodesis $\pm$ interpositional tricortical iliac crest bone graft.

Proximal fixation platform: The talar neck measures 12 to 23 (average, 7) mm with enough room for 1 to 2 screws through a medial column plate without interfering with ankle dorsiflexion.

Distal fixation platform: Inclusion of middle or both middle and lateral cuneiform bones.

- Intercuneiform stabilization. Since the navicular articulates with all 3 cuneiforms, the joint surfaces of each cuneiform are prepared and intercuneiform fixation achieved with a single transverse medial-to-lateral cancellous screw across both inter-cuneiform joints. Alternatively, screws engaging both middle and lateral cuneiform bones through a dorsal plate that straddles both middle and lateral naviculocuneiform joints, will convert the cuneiforms from a mobile segment into a single distal block (Mayich 2016).
- Longitudinal stability. Bicolumnar fixation is preferable to unicolumnar fixation.
- On the medial side where there is nearly always a medial navicular remnant, a single oblique 'longitudinal' screw' engages the medial cuneiform into the talar neck, simulating intramedullary fixation. It is supplemented with a medial column neutralization plate extending from the talus to the navicular (Mayich 2016).
- On the lateral side, where there is nearly always significant bone loss with a defect, tricortical iliac crest bone graft is interposed and held with locking bridging plates.

**Concluding Remarks**

Good surgical planning includes having all anticipated equipment, implants, graft material and biologics available in the operating room. Although it rarely happens, ensure the correct side is checked and marked by the operating surgeon. Visualization of each and every step, from patient positioning to wound closure, will ensure proper execution of the surgical procedure.

The goals are to obtain successful union of arthrodesis sites with a correctly aligned foot. Reduction of medial talonavicular subluxation is important for restoring the medial longitudinal arch and medial column length to minimize risks of nonunion and persistent pain.

## References

Ahmed AA, Kandil MI, Tabl EA, Elgazzar AS. Müller-Weiss disease: a topical review. Foot Ankle Int. 2019;40(12):1447–57. https://doi.org/10.1177/1071100719877000.

Bai W, Li Y, Shen G, et al. Talonavicular-cuneiform arthrodesis for the treatment of Müller-Weiss: mid-term results of 15 cases after 5 years. BMC Musculoskelet Disord. 2023;24:178. https://doi.org/10.1186/s12891-023-06293-1.

Beals TC, Manoli A. The 'peek-a-boo' heel sign in the evaluation of hindfoot varus. Foot. 1996;6(4):205–6. https://doi.org/10.1016/S0958-2592(96)90027-9.

Doyle T, Napier RJ, Wong-Chung J. Recognition and management of Müller-Weiss disease. Foot Ankle Int. 2012;33(4):275–81. https://doi.org/10.3113/FAI.2012.0275.

Li SY, Myerson MS, Monteagudo M, Maceira E. Efficacy of calcaneus osteotomy for treatment of symptomatic Müller-Weiss disease. Foot Ankle Int. 2017;38(3):261–9. https://doi.org/10.1177/1071100716677741.

Mayich, DJ. The treatment of Mueller-Weiss disease: a systematic approach. Tech Foot Ankle Surg. 2016;15(2):59–73. https://doi.org/10.1097/BTF.0000000000000088

Mohiuddin T, Jennison T, Damany D. Müller-Weiss disease—review of current knowledge. Foot Ankle Surg. 2014;20(2):79–84. https://doi.org/10.1016/j.fas.2013.11.001.

Monteagudo M, Maceira E. Management of Müller-Weiss disease. Foot Ankle Clin. 2019;24(1):89–105. https://doi.org/10.1016/j.fcl.2018.09.006.

Sun C, Ebben B, Li S, Zhu M, Myerson MS, Zhang M-Z. The use of SPECT-CT to define treatment for Müller-Weiss disease: a prospective radiographic and clinical study. Foot and Ankle Orthop. 2022;7(4). https://doi.org/10.1177/2473011421S00958

Wong-Chung J, Walls A, Lynch-Wong M, Cassidy R, McKenna R, Wilson A, Stephens M. Towards understanding Müller-Weiss disease from an analysis of 95 cases. Foot Ankle Surg. 2023;29(5):401–11. https://doi.org/10.1016/j.fas.2023.05.004.

# Part II
# Surgery of Müller-Weiss Disease

# Chapter 7
# The Case for Talonaviculocuneiform Arthrodesis

**Abstract** Early studies argued the case against isolated talonavicular or triple arthrodesis in Müller-Weiss disease, as they did not address disease at the naviculocuneiform (NC) articulations and yielded poor outcomes. Instead, they advocated talonaviculocuneiform (TNC) arthrodesis, fusing the talonavicular joint and NC1, and leaving NC2 and NC3 untouched. Others have followed suit, with some adding a reverse V-shaped plantar closing wedge to correct the flattened medial arch. Bony defects resulting from excision of necrotic bone at the lateral navicular are replaced by autogenous tricortical iliac crest bone grafts (TICBG). Some centers deliberately exacerbate the medial talonavicular subluxation and interpose TICBG's between the talar head and middle/lateral cuneiforms bone duo, leaving NC1 out of the fusion mass. Most centers would now include all 3 NC joints. The most rational approach would be to reduce the medial talonavicular subluxation, which is achievable by releasing the medial soft tissues and clearing any obstructions laterally at the 4-corners including the cervical ligament and osteophytes at the calcaneocuboid joint. Consideration should be given to additional calcaneocuboid joint arthrodesis to decrease stress across the TNC arthrodesis and minimize its risk of nonunion.

**Keywords** Müller-Weiss disease · Talonaviculocuneiform arthrodesis · Talonavicular subluxation · Tricortical bone graft · 4-corner release · Calcaneocuboid arthrodesis

## Introduction

Acknowledging that there was no set gold standard for the treatment of Müller-Weiss disease, Fernández de Retana, Maceira et al. (Barcelona, 2004) argued the case against open reduction and internal fixation blaming its poor results to lack of adequate bone stock and presence of osteoarthritis in the perinavicular joints (Fernández de Retana et al. 2004). In their experience, isolated talonavicular arthrodesis yielded moderate outcomes with persistent pain, delayed union and

© The Author(s), under exclusive license to Springer Nature Switzerland AG 2024 
J. Wong-Chung, *Comprehensive Guide to Müller-Weiss Disease*,
https://doi.org/10.1007/978-3-031-66644-5_7

non-union, and did not solve 'incongruence' at the naviculocuneiform joints. Similarly, although union rates were higher with triple arthrodesis, it did not address the naviculocuneiform joints either.

## 7.1 Arthrodesis of Talonavicular and Medial Naviculocuneiform Joints (TNC1)

Therefore instead, the authors advocated talonaviculocuneiform (TNC) arthrodesis using a tricortical bone graft from the iliac crest or proximal tibia without internal fixation. Through a medial approach, a single-piece osteoperiosteal flap was raised off the medial surfaces of the talus, navicular and medial cuneiform bones including the insertion of tibialis posterior tendon. The articular surfaces were prepared. A trough was carved to accept the tricortical bone graft. The foot was plantarflexed to achieve desired arch height. The graft was then locked into place by dorsiflexing the foot, without need for internal fixation. Any residual gaps were filled with cancellous bone chips. The osteoperiosteal flap was replaced and held in position with nonabsorbable sutures.

Although the authors quoted an average follow-up of 6 years, the actual number of operated cases and patient demographics were not specified. Shown as an example, CT scan of one of their patients depicted arthrodesis of the talonavicular and first naviculocuneiform joint. The authors acknowledged that the second and third naviculocuneiform joints were not included in the fusion. They added that this limitation can be addressed through a supplementary dorsolateral approach. They also deemed it unnecessary to include the subtalar joint, because they have not encountered pain at that joint following talonaviculocuneiform arthrodesis alone.

They recognized that talonaviculocuneiform arthrodesis does not address hindfoot varus. Its talonavicular component effectively blocks functional motion at the subtalar joint. Hindfoot varus can hence be corrected by adding a calcaneal slide. Alternatively, by extending the dorsolateral incision into the sinus tarsi, part of the anteromedial portion of the calcaneum is removed and a lever is then used to push the talar head medially, compared to laterally as in progressive collapsing flatfoot deformity. Once the subtalar joint has been everted, a 'calcaneo-stop' screw is inserted at the dorsal non-articular surface of the calcaneus and aimed in a proximal and plantar direction. By leaning it against the lateral surface of the anterior portion of the talus, it acts as a buttress to block the talar head from moving back laterally over the calcaneum.

## 7.2 TNC1 Arthrodesis Incorporating a Reverse V-shaped Osteotomy

Cao HH et al. (Chongqing, China, 2012) echoed the same views as Fernández de Retana et al. (Cao et al. 2012) Through a dorsal approach, they performed TNC1 arthrodesis in 9 feet of 4 men and 5 women, aged 41 to 58 (average, 48.2) years old, with Maceira Stage III disease. MRI scan was obtained preoperatively to assess degree of bone destruction.

After joint preparation, a reverse "V-shaped" plantar closing wedge was removed through the talonavicular joint to restore the medial arch. Using a saw and osteotome, a rectangular trough measuring 3 cm × 1.5 cm × 0.5 cm was then created dorsally extending from the talus to the medial cuneiform. Plantarflexing the forefoot enabled slotting of a tricortical iliac crest bone graft into the trough. It was held in place with 3 cannulated titanium screws directed one each into the talar head, navicular and medial cuneiform bones. As per Fernández de Retana et al., the middle and lateral naviculocuneiform joints were not included in the arthrodesis.

All went on to solid fusion with complete pain relief. Mean AOFAS ankle-hindfoot score improved from 40.1 ± 8.3 preoperatively to 90.9 ± 2.1 at last follow-up.

## 7.3 Arthrodesis of Talonavicular, Middle and Lateral Naviculocuneiform Joints (TNC2-3) with Further Medial Displacement of the Medial Navicular Remnant

Following on along the same lines, Yu et al. (Shanghai, China, 2012) carried out 7 TNC arthrodeses on 6 women and 1 man, aged 46 to 62 (median, 55) years (Yu et al. 2012). The hindfoot was in varus in just 2. The medial arch sagged in 2 feet (Stage IV or V) and the arch was high in only 1 foot (Stage II). But according to Maceira gradings, 4 feet were said to be at Stage III, 1 at Stage IV and 2 at Stage V, with none at Stage II.

A dorsal incision was placed lateral to extensor hallucis longus, which was retracted medially with the neurovascular bundle lying laterally. After joint preparation, a trapezoidal trough was created wider dorsally and narrower plantarwards, except in the 1 foot with pes cavus where a dorsal closing wedge was used to elevate the first ray. Two autogenous tricortical iliac crest bone grafts were fashioned to fit into the bony bed created and held in place with a long Y-shaped plate and screws. Proximally, 3 screws engaged the talar head. Distally, the plate bridged across an unprepared second tarsometatarsal joint. One screw entered the middle cuneiform bone, while 2 distalmost screws engaged the base of the second metatarsal. An additional cancellous lag screw was inserted transversely through the medial navicular remnant into the bone block, with no attempt made to reduce medial subluxation of the talonavicular joint (Fig. 7.1). In the illustration provided, the medial naviculocuneiform (NC1) joint looks unprepared as well as the first intercuneiform joint.

There remains marked persistent medial extrusion of the navicular tuberosity. Except for the one transverse screw across the medial navicular remnant into the bone graft, the first ray appears detached from the second with mobility preserved at NC1 and first intercuneiform joints. No plaster cast was utilized in the postoperative period.

All feet united solidly with an improvement of AOFAS ankle-hindfoot score from 49 preoperatively to 82 at last follow-up. By 2017 and 2018, from the same centre, Zhang and Yu had performed 49 and 69 talonaviculocuneiform arthrodeses, respectively with complete relief of pain and solid fusion in all feet (Zhang and Yu 2017; 2018) .

Although their article title reads 'triple and talonavicular arthrodesis', Lu et al. (Anhui, China, 2022) actually performed talonaviculocuneiform arthrodesis with interpositional tricortical iliac crest bone graft in 12 feet of 8 women and 4 men with an average age of 52.1 years (Lu et al. 2022). According to Maceira's gradings, 7 were at Stage III, 3 at Stage IV and 2 at Stage V.

Their technique is similar to that of Yu (Shanghai, 2012) (Yu et al. 2012; Zhang and Yu 2017, 2018), who is in fact the last-named co-author of Lu's paper. The subtalar and calcaneocuboid joints were said to have been preserved as much as possible, despite the title referring to triple arthrodesis. The written description is equally unclear. After 'thorough loosening of the subtalar, calcaneocuboid and talonavicular joints', the 'navicular bone was completely squeezed out to form a talonavicular or talar wedge joint'. The 'quadrilaterals were straightened out and the force line was corrected in order to restore the arch'.

From the illustrations provided, the subtalar and calcaneocuboid were not prepared or fixed. The lateral two-thirds of the navicular have been excised. A tricortical iliac crest bone graft was interposed between the talar head and middle/lateral cuneiform bone duo. It was held in place by a dorsally placed 6-hole multi-fragment locking plate, with 2 distal screws engaging the middle cuneiform, 2 proximal screws in the talar head and 2 screws in the bone graft. A transverse screw engaged across the medially displaced navicular remnant into the talar head, instead of the bone graft as in Yu's technique (Yu et al. 2012).

Again, no fixation crosses the medial naviculocuneiform joint. No attempt has been made to reduce the medially subluxed navicular. Instead, the medial navicular remnant may have purposefully been 'squeezed out' medially, to create a 'quadrilateral' space for insertion of the tricortical iliac crest bone graft.

All feet united with good pain relief, improvement of function, quality of life and AOFAS score from 43.4 preoperatively to 85.3 at one-year follow-up.

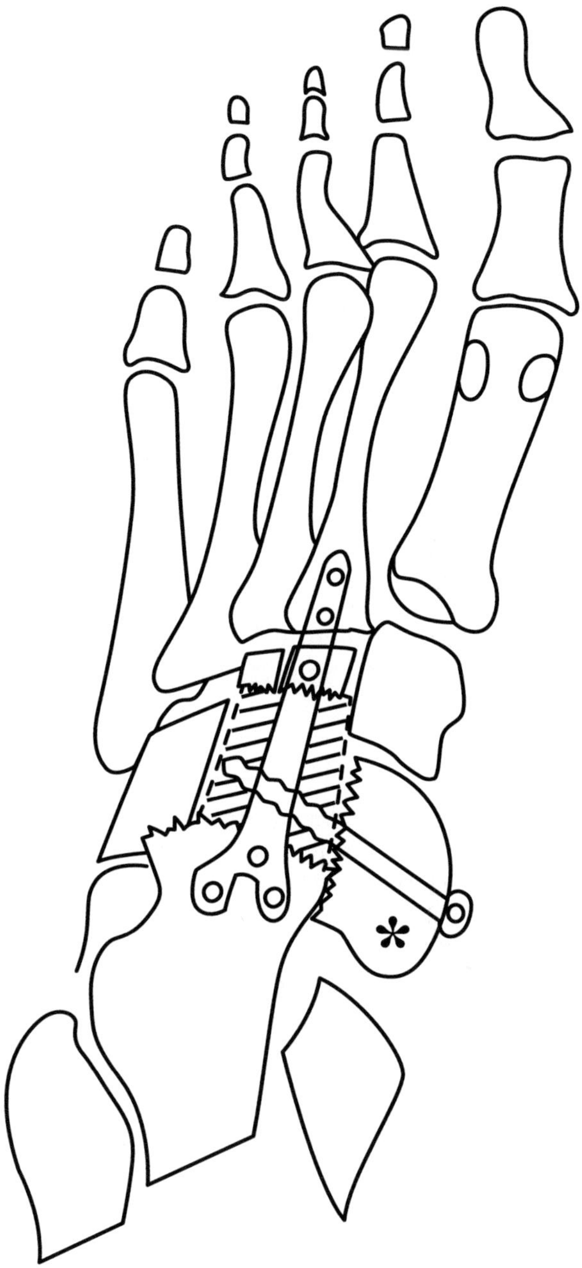


**Fig. 7.1** Schematic representation of technique used by Yu et al. (2012) The avascular lateral portion of the navicular has been excised. The articular surfaces of the talar head, proximal surfaces of the middle and lateral cuneiforms and lateral surface of the medial navicular remnant have been prepared (serrated edges). The medial navicular remnant (*) has been displaced further medially. Two tricortical iliac crest bone grafts (dashed lines surrounding striped area) have been interposed between the middle/lateral cuneiform bone duo and the talar head. A dorsal locking plate bridges the bone graft, with 3 screws engaging the talar head, 1 into the middle cuneiform and 2 across an unprepared second tarsometatarsal joint into the base of the second metatarsal. A separate screw passes transversely across the medial navicular remnant into the bone graft. The medial naviculocuneiform and intercuneiform joints have been left intact

## 7.4 Talonaviculocuneiform Arthrodesis (TNC1-2-3) with Interpositional Tricortical Iliac Crest Bone Graft (TICBG)

Mayich (New Brunswick, Canada, 2016) described his method of talonaviculocuneiform arthrodesis using an interpositional tricortical iliac crest bone graft (TICBG) to replace the avascular lateral part of the navicular (Mayich 2016). The technique is well illustrated on sawbones. The intercuneiform joints are also prepared and a transverse screw traverses the three cuneiform bones from medial to lateral to create a stable distal platform. Another 'longitudinal' screw, which aims to simulate intramedullary fixation, enters the medial cuneiform distally and engages proximally into the talar neck. A dorsomedial plate spans the talonavicular and medial naviculocuneiform joints. A dorsal locking plate bridges over the interpositional TICBG, extending from the lateral talar neck into the middle cuneiform bone.

Despite extensive description of the technique, there is no mention of actual number of cases and operations performed, other than one figure demonstrating postoperative radiographs.

## 7.5 Talonaviculocuneiform Arthrodesis (TNC1-2-3) with TICBG and Reduction of Medial Talonavicular Subluxation

Bai et al. (Guangdong, China, 2023) published their 5-year results of talonaviculocuneiform arthrodesis with interpositional tricortical iliac crest bone graft in 15 feet of 13 women and 2 men, aged 39 to 70 (average, 56) years old (Bai et al. 2023). According to Maceira gradings, 8 were at Stage III and 7 at Stage IV. These 15 were among 84 of 102 feet with Müller-Weiss disease that had undergone surgery. This study from just one centre in China must constitute the second largest series outside of Spain and the biggest series of operated cases in the literature.

The talonavicular and naviculocuneiform joints are exposed through a dorsal approach. Using sharp dissection, the navicular is freed medially by releasing the plantar soft tissues including the plantar ligament, leaving only the attachment of tibialis posterior tendon. Laterally, the '4-corners' as termed by Doyle et al. (2012) is debrided. It is the junction between the inferolateral border of the talar head, lateral corner of the navicular, anterior process of the calcaneum and adjoining superior border of the cuboid. It is contiguous with the anterior facet of the subtalar joint.

With compression and fragmentation of the plantar and lateral navicular, its medial half rotates internally leading to shortening of the medial column. The talar head moves laterally and plantarwards, pressing against the anterior calcaneal process. Heel varus and paradoxical pes planus varus ensue with transfer of forefoot forces to the lateral midfoot. Degenerative changes develop with osteophyte formation at the calcaneocuboid joint and the '4-corners'.

To obtain reduction of the navicular, Bai et al. emphasize the importance of débridement of the '4-corners'. Resection of osteophytes at the anterolateral border of the talar head enables reduction of the talonavicular joint in the sagittal plane. Release of the cervical ligament at the anterior aspect of the sinus tarsi and excision of osteophyte around the calcaneocuboid joint allows adduction and internal rotation of the talar head in the transverse plane.

Following joint preparation, the navicular is reduced from its subluxed medial and plantar location using a periosteal elevator to push and rotate it lateralward and dorsalward to its correct position at the apex of the medial arch. Reduction is held with two to three temporary K-wires. Correction of the medial longitudinal arch and talonavicular reduction are verified under image intensifier. All lateral necrotic bone is then excised. Using an osteotome, a bony trough is created. In the longitudinal axis, its bed is rectangular. In the mediolateral plane, its roof is trapezoidal with a wider lateral base. The tricortical iliac crest bone graft is fashioned and inserted into the gap thus created between the talar head and lateral cuneiforms. Fixation is obtained with 2 cannulated lag screws across the medial and middle talonaviculocuneiform joints (TNC1 and TNC2) and a dorsal locking plate spanning TNC2 and TNC3. Where required, an additional Herbert screw is inserted transversely to stabilize the bone block to the medial navicular remnant (Fig. 7.2A–B).

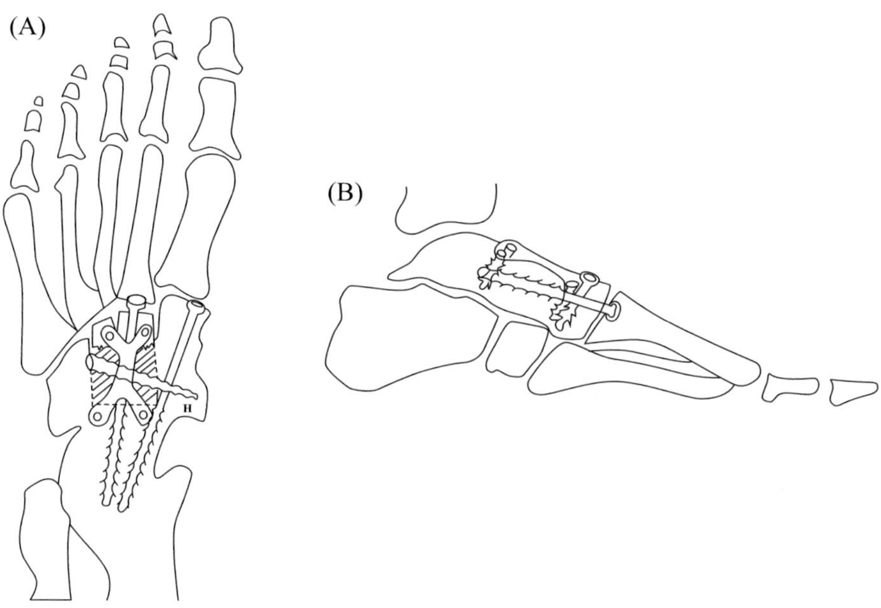


**Fig. 7.2** Schematic representation of fixation technique used by Bai et al. (A) Striped area represents tricortical iliac crest bone graft. Following reduction of the talonavicular subluxation, 2 screws engage the medial and intermediate cuneiforms distally across the medial navicular remnant and bone graft into the talar head proximally. One screw each engages the medial and lateral distal screw holes of a dorsal X-locking plate into the intermediate and lateral cuneiforms, respectively. An additional transverse Herbert screw (H) stabilizes the graft to the medial navicular remnant. (B) Lateral projection

The authors report no delayed or nonunion with their technique. Mean AOFAS scores increased by 48.67 while median VAS score decreased by 6. Calcaneal pitch, talonavicular coverage, Kite's angle, lateral and dorsoplantar talo-first metatarsal angles all improved significantly ($p < 0.05$).

Several important points are worth elaborating upon. The authors recognize that length of the medial column should be restored. However, they rightly believe that it is far more important to reduce the medial talonavicular subluxation, as it is the main factor contributing to relative shortening of the medial column. Laterally rotating the navicular bone back to its normal position at the apex of the medial longitudinal arch automatically restores length of the medial column while simultaneously correcting the medial longitudinal arch. Reduction of the medial talonavicular subluxation is a prerequisite as it also prepares the scene for reconstruction of the lateral talus-navicular-cuneiform column.

This approach stands in complete contrast to that of Yu (2012) and Lu (2022), where the medial navicular remnant appears to have been intentionally displaced even further medially to create a 'quadrilateral' space for the interpositional tricortical iliac crest bone graft, thus exacerbating the medial prominence caused by the navicular tuberosity. The prominence of the medially extruded navicular tuberosity itself is a frequent cause of complaint before surgery, and often after surgery if medial talonavicular subluxation has not been reduced. To further displace the navicular tuberosity medially is likely to create further symptoms medially. Therefore, besides the biomechanical correction it brings about, reduction of medial talonavicular subluxation also eliminates the troublesome prominence of the navicular tuberosity.

Bai et al. advised against triple arthrodesis as recommended by some authors for Maceira Stages IV and V disease. They believe that fusion of the subtalar and calcaneocuboid joints is not only unnecessary but also causes hindfoot stiffness and decreases foot function. They affirm that the talonavicular and naviculocuneiform joints are the joints primarily involved in the pathological process, whereas the subtalar and calcaneocuboid joints are secondary sites.

Although degeneration was present preoperatively at the calcaneocuboid and subtalar joints in 53.3% and 20% respectively, none were tender over these two joints, which were therefore not included in the arthrodesis. Post-operatively, none had further progression of degeneration at these 2 joints, which remained asymptomatic. The authors concluded that talonaviculocuneiform arthrodesis with interpositional tricortical iliac crest bone graft may delay or halt the progression of arthritis at the calcaneocuboid and subtalar joints.

In one patient with persistent lateral forefoot pain with callosity over the base of the fifth metatarsal at 4 years following talonaviculocuneiform arthrodesis, residual forefoot supination and heel varus were deemed to be the cause. Midfoot derotational osteotomy combined with lateral displacement calcaneal osteotomy resolved her pain.

## 7.6 Talonaviculocuneiform Arthrodesis with Reduction of Medial Talonavicular Subluxation—Case Report

Nelson and Rivello (California, USA, 2012) reported on a 28-year-old healthy Hispanic woman with 'unilateral tarsal scaphoiditis' treated successfully by talonaviculocuneiform arthrodesis (Nelson and Rivello 2012). The technical difficulties encountered during surgery are worth elaborating upon.

The patient, whose BMI was 25, gave a two-years' history of pain and swelling over the dorsum of the right midfoot. Dorsoplantar radiograph showed compression of the lateral half of the navicular, degenerative changes more marked at the talonavicular than at the naviculocuneiform joints, a short first metatarsal and a positive cuboid sign. Lateral radiograph demonstrated sagging at the talonavicular joint, dorsal osteophyte at the talar head and a wide-open sinus tarsi. CT scan revealed a dorsally extruded fragment that 'appeared to articulate with both the talus and the tarsal navicular'. Features were deemed consistent with Müller-Weiss disease – Wong Group 3B Maceira Stage V. A custom-made ankle–foot orthotic brace did not relieve her pain. Based upon advice obtained at a North American AO conference, surgery was embarked upon.

Initial approach was dorsal between the anterior tibial and extensor hallucis longus tendons. Despite releasing soft tissues around the dorsal aspect of the talar neck, navicular and cuneiforms, the talonavicular joint could not be reduced. Extensive scar tissue laterally and contracture of ligaments at the subtalar joint were thought to be preventing reduction. A second 8-cm incision was made extending from the tip of the fibula to the base of the fourth metatarsal to expose the sinus tarsi. The interosseous and cervical ligaments were sharply divided. The calcaneocuboid joint, exposed by reflecting the extensor digitorum brevis muscle distally, appeared normal.

The extruded lateral navicular fragment, which constituted 30 to 40% of total navicular volume, was excised. A peculiar facet was noted between the anterior calcaneal process and talar head and neck. It was thought to have resulted from longstanding deformity. The lateral margin of the talus was released to allow motion between the talus and calcaneus. A Cobb elevator was introduced along the peculiar facet to allow for leverage of the anterior and medial margin of the talar head, which lay displaced laterally in the center of the foot. To effect reduction, pressure was applied to the lateral part of the talar head pushing it medialward, while simultaneous pressure was applied lateralward to the medial navicular remnant.

Fixation was obtained with a 7.3 mm cannulated screw inserted over a guide wire at the medial cuneiform across the navicular into the talar body. A trough was created for an inlay graft extending from the talar neck across the medial navicular remnant to the base of the medial and intermediate cuneiform bones. A tricortical iliac crest allograft was slotted into the trough and stabilized with two 4.0 mm cancellous lag screws, one engaging the lateral talar neck proximally and the other distally into the middle cuneiform (Fig. 7.3A–B).

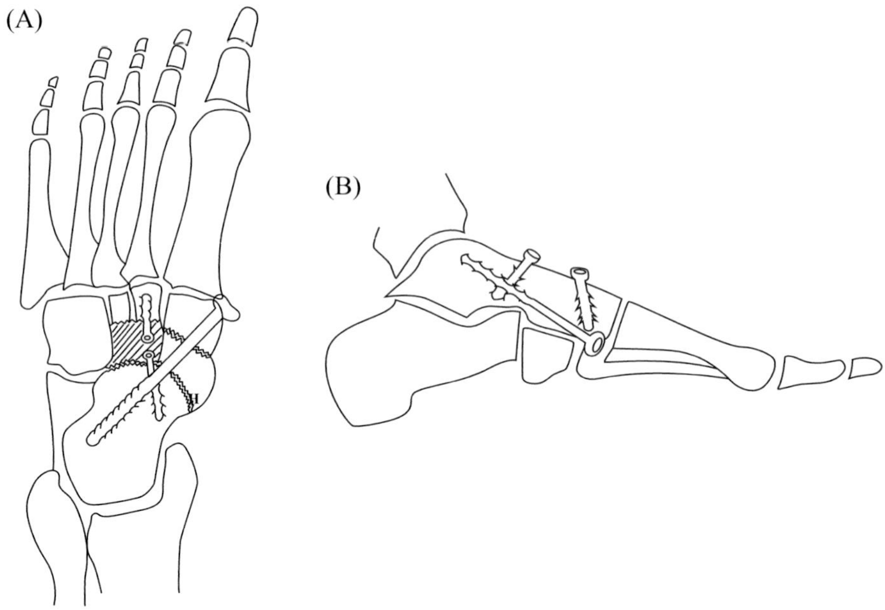


**Fig. 7.3** Schematic representation of fixation technique used by Nelson and Rivolli. (A) Serrated edges denote joint preparation. Striped area represents bone graft. One lag screw enters the medial cuneiform bone distally across the medial naviculocuneiform and talonavicular joints into the talar head. One screw each stabilizes the bone graft to the talar head proximally and the middle cuneiform distally. (B) Lateral projection

At final follow-up of 38 months, the talonaviculocuneiform arthrodesis had united solidly. The patient reported significant pain relief with improvement of ankle hindfoot score from 32 to 97.

To some extent, the surgical technique resembles that of Bai et al., in that both recommend clearance of blockages at the lateral corner of the navicular (Bai et al. 2023).

## 7.7 Talonaviculocuneiform Arthrodesis with Reduction of Medial Talonavicular Subluxation—Example

This section exemplifies reduction of marked medial talonavicular subluxation in a 64-year-old woman from the series of Wong-Chung et al. (2024) Radiographs demonstrated concomitant severe compression of the lateral navicular and lateral naviculocuneiform joints (Fig. 7.4A–C). The second metatarsal is much longer than the first. Except for midfoot abduction in her case, the radiographic features are identical to those shown in the seventh illustration of Harnroongroj and Chuckpaiwong (2018). In view of the marked radiographic changes, inflammatory markers, glucose profile and nerve conduction studies were obtained to exclude a neuropathic condition. All proved normal including a thorough neurological assessment. Interestingly, Brailsford's series in 1939 also included cases with marked medial talonavicular subluxation approaching near to complete dislocation (Brailsford 1939).

The medial navicular remnant was displaced medially and plantarward, whereas the talar head had shifted laterally to lie in the midline of the foot. Medial soft tissue release and lateral clearance were performed to enable reduction of the talonavicular articulation. After joint preparation, more than a third of the lateral navicular was deemed not substantial enough to secure bony union (Fig. 7.4D). It was excised and replaced with an interpositional tricortical iliac crest bone graft. The first, second and third tarsometatarsal (TMT) joints were also prepared and included in the fusion mass.

Postoperative radiographs show the medial navicular remnant has been reduced to its correct position at the apex of the medial arch. Medial column length and height have been restored. Screw fixation is similar to that of Nelson and Rivello (2012), except that it was inserted in antegrade instead of retrograde fashion (Figs. 7.3, 7.4). Proximally, it engaged the posterolateral corner of the talus. Distally, it extended across the medial navicular remnant, middle and medial cuneiform bones and a prepared TMT1 into the base of the first metatarsal for better purchase (Fig. 7.4E–G). A tricortical iliac crest bone graft was inserted between the talar head and middle/lateral cuneiform bone duo instead of an inlay graft. It was held in position by 2 bridging plates extending from the talar head across the prepared TMT2 and TMT3. The author would have been preferred medial column plating rather than this simulated form of intramedullary screw fixation. It was not available at the time, which illustrates the importance of having the necessary equipment and implants in the operating room as recommended by Mayich et al. (2016)

This case serves to reinforce the concept shared by Bai et al. (2023), Nelson et al. ( 2012) and Yuan et al. (2019), that it is possible to reduce even severe degrees of medial talonavicular subluxation. Fusion, in-situ or with imperfect reduction, would have left a permanent deformity and not resolved her foot problem in the long term. Reduction of medial talonavicular subluxation is preferable to in-situ arthrodesis.

## 7.8 Talonaviculocuneiform (TNC1-2-3) Plus Calcaneocuboid Arthrodesis

Ahmad (Philadelphia, USA, 2015) described his philosophy of perinavicular arthrodesis for advanced osteonecrosis of the navicular (Ahmad 2015). The introduction discusses aetiology and treatment of Müller-Weiss disease in detail. The results section refers to treatment of 10 feet with Müller-Weiss disease in 7 women and 3 men aged 34 to 70 (mean, 55) years old. However, causes of osteonecrosis were said to have included trauma in 3, sickle-cell anemia in 2 and oral steroids in 2. Perhaps the other 3 feet might have been cases of Müller-Weiss disease. The first

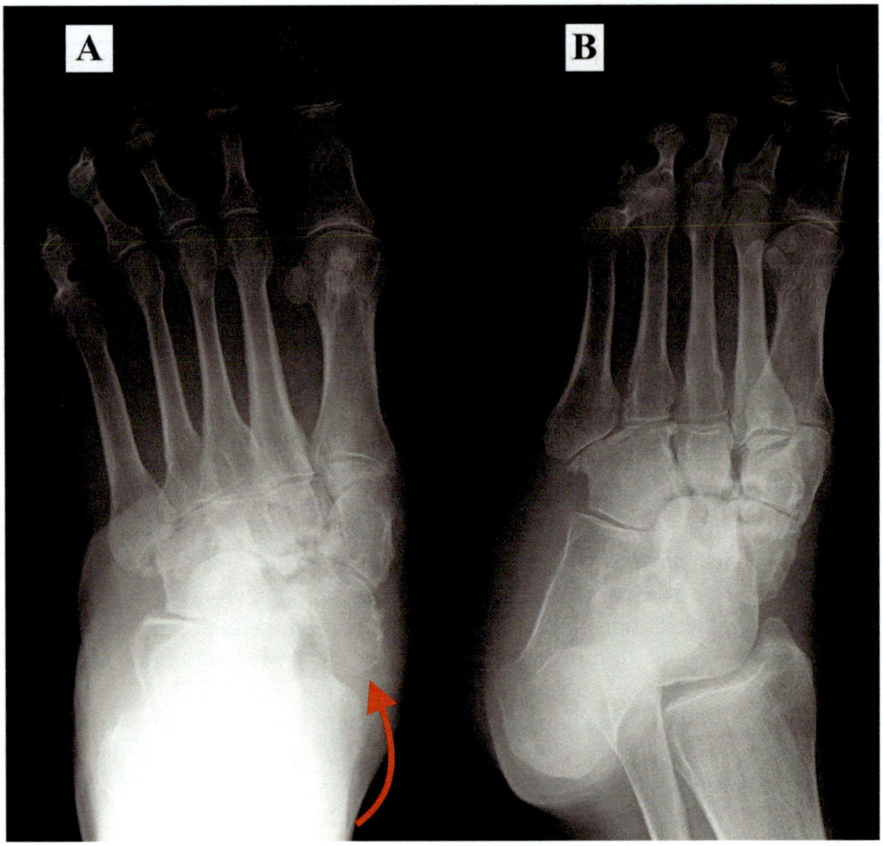


**Fig. 7.4** (A) Dorsoplantar (B) medial oblique and (C) lateral standing radiographs of the left foot and ankle of a 64-year-old woman with normal neurology, inflammatory markers, glucose profile and nerve conduction studies. Note the overlong second metatarsal. Compression changes at the lateral navicular and naviculocuneiform joints. Marked medial talonavicular subluxation and medial extrusion of navicular pole. Talar head shifted laterally to lie in midline of the foot. Medial navicular remnant markedly displaced medially and plantarwards with shortening of the medial column and midfoot abduction as shown by a negative dorsoplantar talo-first metatarsal angle. Red arrows indicate direction of corrective force. (D) Intraoperative photograph of the left foot following joint preparation of the talonavicular and naviculocuneiform joints. Toes are covered with blue adhesive drape, retractor at lateral side and bone lever medially. Red rubber loop around neurovascular bundle. Following medial soft tissue release and lateral clearance, the navicular has been reduced from its displaced medial and plantar location to its normal correct position at the apex of the medial arch. The lateral third or more of the navicular was considered too insubstantial for guaranteed union. It was excised and replaced with an interpositional tricortical iliac crest bone graft. The first, second and third tarsometatarsal joints were also prepared and included in the fusion. (E–G) Talonaviculocuneiform arthrodesis was stabilized with an antegrade 6.7 mm lag screw (Arthrex Inc., Naples, FL) inserted at the posterolateral corner of the talus, across the medial navicular remnant, intermediate and medial cuneiforms into the base of the first metatarsal. Two dorsal locking plates bridged over the bone graft from the talar head into the base of the second and third metatarsals (VariAx, Stryker Leibinger GmbH & Co, Freiburg, Germany)

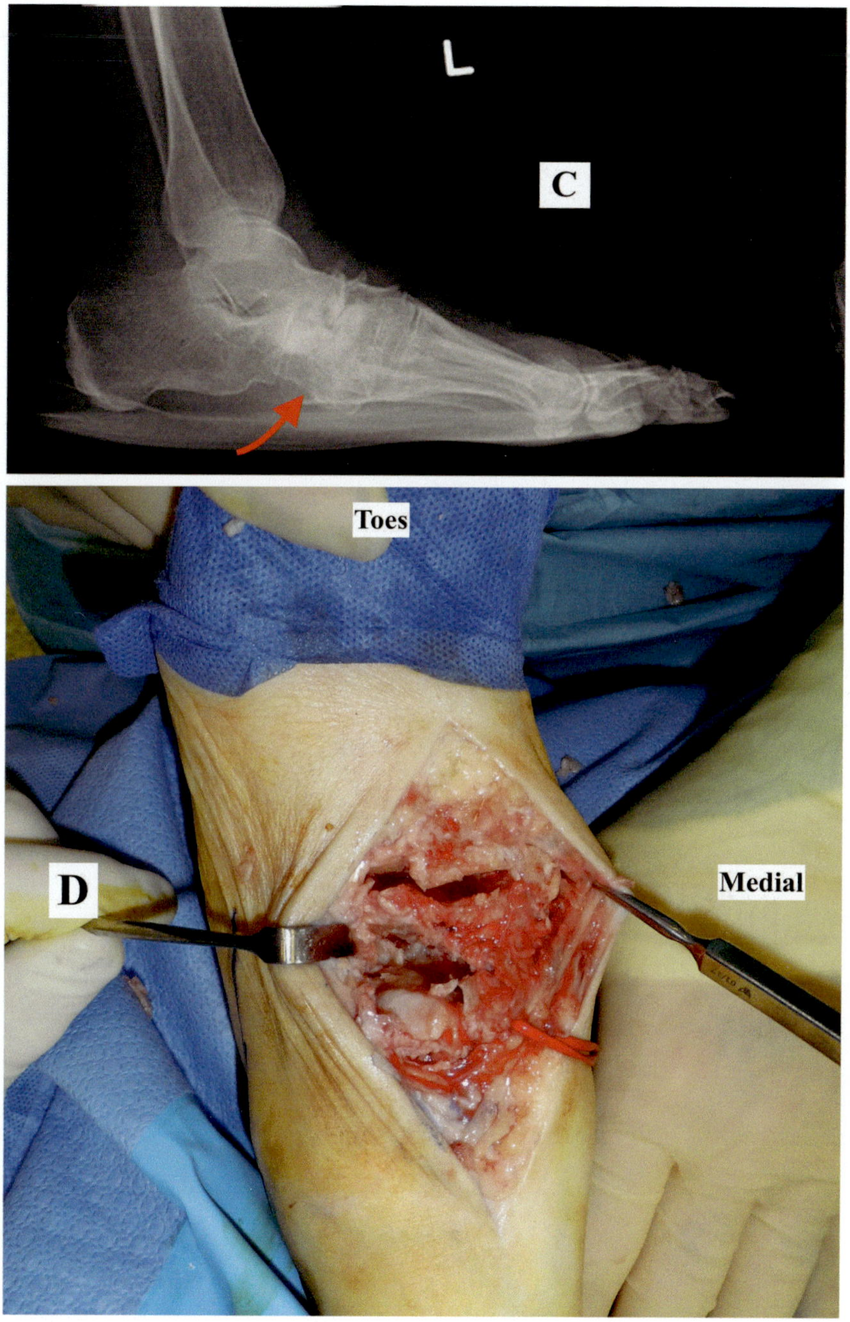


**Fig. 7.4** (continued)

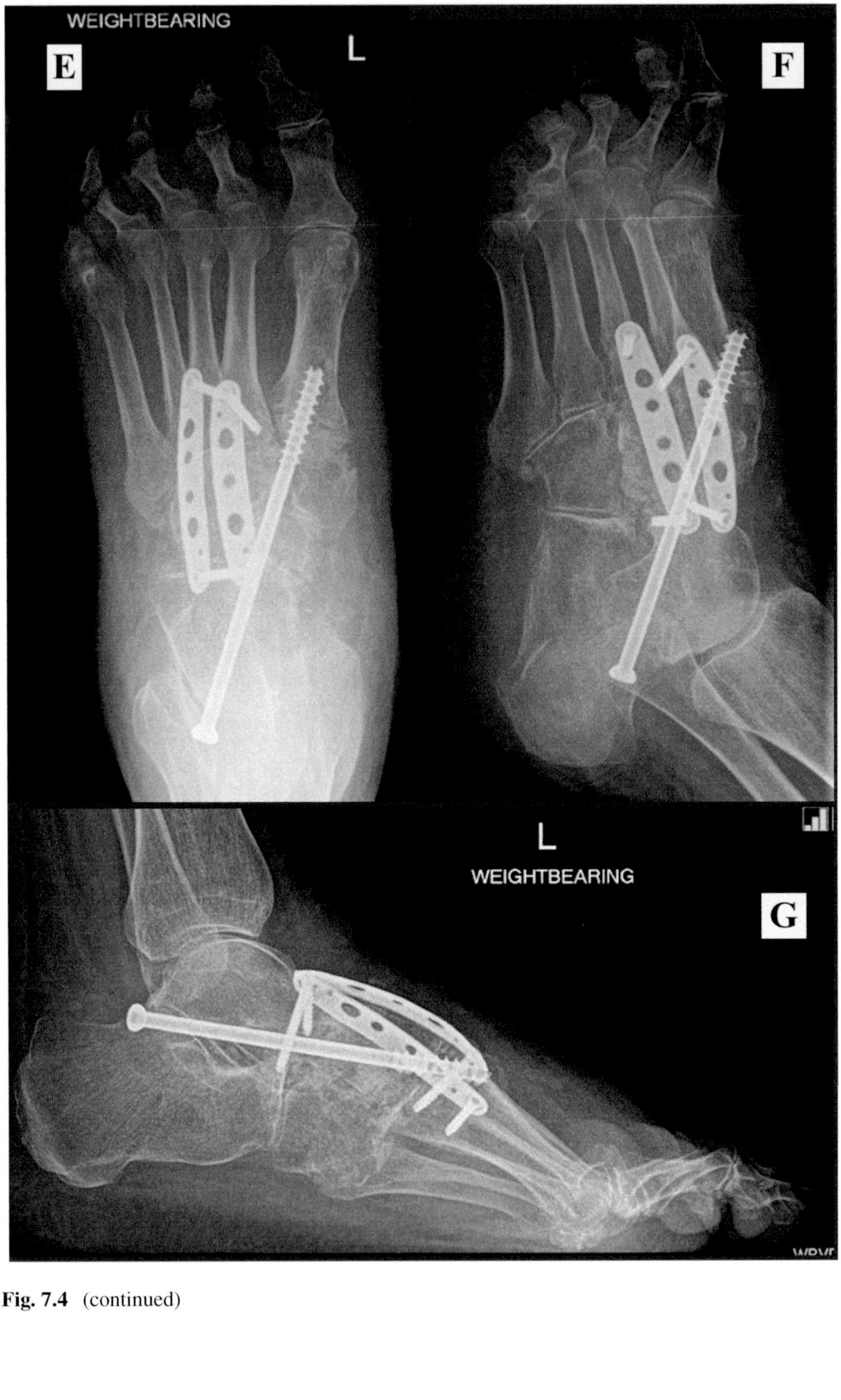


Fig. 7.4 (continued)

illustration depicts a comma-shaped left navicular with compression more marked at the naviculocuneiform side, midfoot abduction and minimal medial talonavicular subluxation. These features are consistent with a Group 3C reverse Müller-Weiss pattern. The second plain radiographic illustration purports to show Müller-Weiss disease. However, there is impression of generalized extensive necrosis throughout the navicular. The third illustration shows just one sagittal MRI slice of a foot diagnosed as having Müller-Weiss disease.

Nevertheless, the article raises certain very pertinent points. Besides not addressing disease at the naviculocuneiform joint, isolated talonavicular arthrodesis is prone to nonunion due to high stresses, as long as the calcaneocuboid joint remains mobile. Likewise, although talonaviculocuneiform arthrodesis addresses disease at the naviculocuneiform joint, it also remains exposed to significant stress in the presence of a mobile calcaneocuboid joint. Ahmad therefore advocates a 'perinavicular' arthrodesis of the talonavicular, all 3 naviculocuneiform and the calcaneocuboid joints supplemented with structural autologous iliac crest bone graft to replace all necrotic bone and reinforced by cancellous iliac crest bone chips.

He obtains an MRI as part of the preoperative planning to quantify the amount of necrotic bone. The patient is positioned supine with a bump beneath the ipsilateral buttock to bring the foot into a straight upright position. The ipsilateral pelvis is prepped for harvesting iliac crest bone. Dual surgical approaches consist of a dorsal incision between tibialis anterior and extensor hallucis tendons, and a lateral incision extending from the tip of the fibula to the fourth tarsometatarsal joint. Distal reflection of the extensor digitorum brevis muscle belly exposes the calcaneocuboid joint.

Excision of the navicular is said to range from partial to complete 'naviculectomy'. Deformity correction is obtained by combined eversion of the transverse tarsal joints and plantarflexion of the first ray. If there is no heel varus or gapping at the calcaneocuboid joint, it is fused in situ. Any residual hindfoot varus is corrected by shortening the lateral column through the calcaneocuboid joint. Fixation is obtained using a dorsal H-shaped plate and screw construct (ALPS, Biomet, Warsaw, IN)) and compression staples laterally.

Except for 1 delayed union, all went on to full radiological union at a mean of 16.8 weeks. Mean VAS scores decreased from 8.2 to 1.3 ($p < 0.001$) while Foot and Ankle Disability Measures—Activities of Daily Living increased from 34% to 91.2% ($p < 0.05$). No patient had developed adjacent joint arthritis at last follow-up.

Although Ahmad considers Köhler's disease as a different entity, he may have assumed the term Müller-Weiss disease encompasses all forms of osteonecrosis, regardless of cause. This may explain why some of his cases required complete 'naviculectomy', since it is rare for the whole navicular to be completely necrotic in Müller-Weiss disease. Regarding the technical tip, other surgeons have also highlighted the need to include the calcaneocuboid joint when performing talonavicular or naviculocuneiform arthrodesis (Clain and Baxter 1994; Haddad 2019). Wong-Chung et al. included the calcaneocuboid joint when performing talonavicular arthrodesis in Feet 25 and 31 (Wong-Chung et al. 2024). However, they subsequently opted to preserve the calcaneocuboid joint and performed double medial instead of triple arthrodesis.

### Concluding Remarks

Talonaviculocuneiform (TNC) arthrodesis was initially advocated as the surgery of choice for Müller-Weiss disease, because talonavicular fusion did not address pathology at the naviculocuneiform (NC) articulation.

Variations in the procedure include (i) addition of a plantar closing wedge osteotomy through the talonavicular articulation, (ii) fusing NC1 alone leaving NC2 and NC3 untouched (TNC1), (iii) exacerbating the medial talonavicular subluxation by displacing the navicular tuberosity further medially and interposing a tricortical iliac crest bone graft between the talar head and the intermediate and lateral cuneiform bones (TNC2-3). Most centers would include all 3 NC joints in the fusion mass (TNC1-2-3).

Talonaviculocuneiform arthrodesis is indicated for disease affecting both talonavicular and naviculocuneiform joints. For best results, it is preferable to reduce the medial talonavicular subluxation by medial soft tissue release and lateral clearance of obstructions at the 4-corners. Relocating the navicular from a medial and plantar displaced location to its normal position at the apex of the medial arch automatically restores medial column length and medial arch height.

## References

Ahmad J. Perinavicular arthrodesis as treatment of advanced navicular osteonecrosis. Tech Foot Ankle Surg. 2015;14:79–87. https://doi.org/10.1097/BTF.0000000000000090.

Bai W, Li Y, Shen G, Zhang H, Li X, Zhu Y. Talonavicular-cuneiform arthrodesis for the treatment of Müller-Weiss: mid-term results of 15 cases after 5 years. BMC Musculoskelet Disord. 2023;24:178. https://doi.org/10.1186/s12891-023-06293-1.

Brailsford JF. Osteochondritis of the adult tarsal navicular. J Bone Joint Surg. 1939;21(1):111–20.

Cao HH, Tang KL, Xu JZ. Peri-navicular arthrodesis for the stage III Müller-Weiss disease. Foot Ankle Int. 2012;33(6):475–8. https://doi.org/10.3113/FAI.2012.0475.

Clain MR, Baxter DE. Simultaneous calcaneocuboid and talonavicular fusion. Long-term follow-up study. J Bone Joint Surg Br. 1994;76(1):133–6.

Doyle T, Napier RJ, Wong-Chung J. Recognition and management of Müller-Weiss disease. Foot Ankle Int. 2012;33(4):275–81. https://doi.org/10.3113/FAI.2012.0275.

Fernández de Retana P, Maceira E, Fernández-Valencia JA, Suso S. Arthrodesis of the talonavicular-cuneiform joints in Müller-Weiss disease. Foot Ankle Clin. 2004;9(1):65–72. https://doi.org/10.1016/S1083-7515(03)00175-X

Haddad SL. Using calcaneocuboid fusion to your advantage. Advanced surgical techniques in foot and ankle reconstruction: beyond basic procedures. *AOFAS* Hands-on Course, Orthopaedic Learning Center, Illinois. Sep 2019.

Harnroongroj T, Chuckpaiwong B. Müller-Weiss disease: three- to eight-year follow-up outcomes of isolated talonavicular arthrodesis. J Foot Ankle Surg. 2018;57(5):1014–9. https://doi.org/10.1053/j.jfas.2018.01.008.

Lu L, Liu B, Zeng J, Chen W, Hu F, Ma Q, Yu G. Efficacy of triple and talonavicular arthrodesis for the treatment of III-V Müller-Weiss disease. Tohoku J Exp Med. 2022;258(2):97–102. https://doi.org/10.1620/tjem.2022.J062.

Mayich DJ. The treatment of Mueller-Weiss disease: a systematic approach. Tech Foot Ankle Surg. 2016;15(2):59–73. https://doi.org/10.1097/BTF.0000000000000088.

Nelson EW, Rivello GJ. Müller-Weiss disease of the tarsal navicular: an idiopathic case. J Foot Ankle Surg. 2012;51(5):636–41. https://doi.org/10.1053/j.jfas.2012.04.002.

Wong-Chung J, Blythe A, Lynch-Wong M, McKenna R, Wilson A, Stephens M. Outcomes of selective arthrodesis based on joints affected in 33 feet with Müller-Weiss disease. J Foot Ankle Surg. 2024;63(2):199–206. https://doi.org/10.1053/j.jfas.2023.11.001

Yu G, Zhao Y, Zhou J, Zhang M. Fusion of talonavicular and naviculocuneiform joints for the treatment of Müller-Weiss disease. J Foot Ankle Surg. 2012;51(4):415–9. https://doi.org/10.1053/j.jfas.2012.04.004.

Yuan C, Wang C, Zhang C, Huang J, Wang X, Ma X. Derotation of the talus and arthrodesis treatment of stages II-V Müller-Weiss disease: midterm results of 36 cases. Foot Ankle Int. 2019;40(5):506–14. https://doi.org/10.1177/1071100719829457.

Zhang MZ, Yu GR. Surgical treatment for Müller-Weiss disease. Foot Ankle Orthop. 2017;2(3). https://doi.org/10.1177/2473011417S000430

Zhang MZ, Yu GR. Surgical treatment for Müller-Weiss disease. Foot Ankle Orthop. 2018;3(3). https://doi.org/10.1177/2473011418S00536

# Chapter 8
# The Case for Joint-Preserving Surgery

**Abstract** Core decompression is indicated when the disease occasionally presents at Maceira stage I with no bony abnormality detectable on plain radiographs. Based on the notion of mandatory heel varus, some centers advocate lateral displacement calcaneal osteotomy only in Müller-Weiss disease, preserving all the diseased midfoot joints. Should this joint-preserving surgery fail, arthrodesis can always be performed later with the added advantage of heel varus having already been corrected by calcaneal osteotomy. On a cautionary note, the presence of heel varus should be verified preoperatively by obtaining a hindfoot alignment radiograph. Contrary to the previous approach, Egyptian adolescents underwent calcaneal lengthening instead to simultaneously correct flatfoot and midfoot abduction. Geographical differences may exist that deserve further investigation.

**Keywords** Müller-Weiss disease · Core decompression · Heel varus · Calcaneal osteotomy · Lateral column lengthening · Midfoot abduction

### Introduction

Patients always prefer joint-preserving surgery whenever possible. Surgeons will always attempt joint-preserving surgery wherever possible.

## 8.1 Core Decompression for Stage I Müller-Weiss Disease

According to Maceira's classification, Stage I represents the earliest stage of Müller-Weiss disease with no abnormality detectable on plain radiographs. Diagnosis is made by MRI or scintigraphy. Although in practice most patients present with established degeneration and deformity, there have been case reports on use of core decompression in Stage I disease (Janositz et al. 2011; Fontaine et al. 1948).

© The Author(s), under exclusive license to Springer Nature Switzerland AG 2024

J. Wong-Chung, *Comprehensive Guide to Müller-Weiss Disease*,
https://doi.org/10.1007/978-3-031-66644-5_8

Janositz et al. (Hungary, 2010) reported on an 18-year-old athlete who presented with left foot pain (Janositz et al. 2011). Plain radiographs showed no bony abnormality. Tc-99m HDP bone scintigraphy demonstrated increased activity during the perfusion, blood-pool and metabolic phases. MRI revealed altered signal intensity in the proximal and dorsal part of the navicular. After 4 months of failed nonoperative treatment, she underwent percutaneous core decompression using a 3.2 mm drill bit via dorsomedial and dorsolateral drill holes. Three months later, she was pain-free and returned to competitive sports winning medals. Repeat MRI at 8 years' follow-up showed complete return to normal of bone marrow signal.

There is no mention of metatarsal lengths. Signal intensity was altered in the dorsal and proximal part of the navicular, whereas compression usually affects the plantar and lateral part of the bone.

## 8.2 "Super" Lateral Displacement Calcaneal Osteotomy (LDCO)

On the one hand, Fernández de Retana, Maceira et al. (Spain, 2004) had argued the case and set the pace for talonaviculocuneiform arthrodesis in the surgical treatment of Müller-Weiss disease (Fernández de Retana et al. 2004). In 2008, Li, Myerson, Monteagudo and Maceira initiated a complete trend reversal aiming instead to save all the foot joints with their novel approach of a "super" lateral displacement and lateral closing wedge calcaneal osteotomy (Avila et al. 2016; Li et al. 2016, 2017).

The rationale behind this strategy is based primarily upon the premise of heel varus as a hallmark deformity, Maceira having previously coined the term 'paradoxical pes planus varus' in Müller-Weiss disease (Maceira and Rochera 2004). To support their approach, the authors cited Hetsroni et al., who had compared pedobarographic measurements in 8 feet with Müller-Weiss disease against 18 normal feet (Hetsroni et al. 2007). Hetsroni et al. (Israel, 2007) had noted significantly lower pressures in the medial heel segments ($p = 0.015$), besides significantly higher pressures in the midfoot segments ($p < 0.05$) and lower pressures in the toes ($p < 0.01$) of feet with Müller-Weiss disease. They had assessed heel position clinically without confirmation by radiographic hindfoot alignment views. Clinically then, the diseased feet had a mean standing heel varus angle of 5° compared to a mean heel valgus of 5° in the control group. Maceira gradings were not listed, although all feet were said to have advanced radiographic characteristics. Their illustration depicted a case of Group 3B Maceira Stage V, involving the talonavicular more than the naviculocuneiform joints with the talar head articulating directly with the lateral cuneiform.

In further support of their approach, Li et al. (2017) quoted Lui who felt that one of his 6 patients, who complained of persistent lateral foot pain following arthroscopic triple arthrodesis and had increased lateral sole pressure on pedobarography, would have benefited from a lateral displacement calcaneal osteotomy (Lui 2009). Monteagudo and Maceira had also noticed that patients who had undergone arthrodesis fared better with lower complication rates including of talonavicular nonunion, if hindfoot varus had been corrected (Monteagudo and Maceira 2019).

Li et al. remarked that not all feet with Müller-Weiss disease require surgery despite the presence of advanced osteoarthritis. Symptoms can be quite minimal, can remain subtle for many years and may not correspond with pathoradiological changes.

They had also observed that 80% of their cases showed symptomatic improvement with a lateral heel wedge and a medial arch support. They inferred that there must be some degree of motion remaining in the perinavicular joint complex so that the orthotic can cause the talus to move medially over the calcaneus, thereby shifting compressive forces from the diseased cartilage at the lateral navicular to the healthier cartilage of the medial navicular.

The authors undertook a retrospective multicentre study of 14 feet in 7 women and 6 men with an average age of 56 (range, 33–79) years. Their stated criterion for inclusion was an initial positive response to a rigid orthotic consisting of a medial arch support with the heel posted in valgus. Six patients expressed reluctance to wear the orthosis indefinitely. Seven had a limited response to the orthotic but wished to avoid arthrodesis. Yet, patients were said to have been excluded if they had long-lasting improvement from the support or if the orthotic gave no benefit at all, in which case they proceeded to arthrodesis. According to Maceira's classification, 5 feet were at Stage II, 4 at Stage III, 4 at Stage IV and 1 at Stage V. All patients had heel varus clinically. Saltzman's hindfoot alignment views were obtained in all, but no values were given.

Surgery consisted of a combination of a laterally based closing wedge osteotomy of 5 mm and a lateral calcaneal slide of 3–4 mm, with no other associated procedures. Results were excellent in 4, good in 8 and fair in 2 cases with no poor outcome. All patients improved significantly with no worsening of arthritis or stage of disease. Maceira stage did not influence clinical outcome, with all feet benefiting whatever their stage. None required conversion to arthrodesis at an average follow-up of 3.7 (range, 1–8.5) years.

On a more cautious note, the authors advised informing patients that calcaneal osteotomy is worthwhile trying, but that it may not work, in which case secondary arthrodesis can still be performed. Nor is it possible to predict if an arthrodesis will be necessary in future. The authors acknowledged the limitations of a small number of cases with no control group, the lack of clear understanding as to how LDCO alleviates symptoms and their assumption that changes in forces occur around the perinavicular joints solely by inference from postoperative clinical and radiological appearances.

Of note, their illustration of a foot with adult-onset Group 3B (TN > NC) Maceira Stage IV disease that underwent lateral displacement calcaneal osteotomy clearly shows the heel to be offset in valgus and not in varus on preoperative hindfoot alignment radiograph. On lateral standing radiographs, the arch sags by a measurable 4° at the naviculocuneiform joint post calcaneal osteotomy compared to a neutral Méary's angle preoperatively.

In 2019, Monteagudo and Maceira reported that one of their 18 patients necessitated conversion to talonaviculocuneiform arthrodesis 4 years after calcaneal osteotomy. Surgery was said to be easier as previous heel varus had already been corrected. Further along the article, another patient is said to have undergone conversion to triple arthrodesis also 4 years later (Monteagudo and Maceira 2019).

They showed examples of 2 feet, in which the lateral talonavicular joint space improved following calcaneal osteotomy, purportedly due to medial shift of the talar head. They go further to state that even patients, who do not respond positively to a lateral heel wedge and medial arch support, benefit from calcaneal osteotomy (unpublished data). Encouraged by their experience, calcaneal osteotomy is now their surgical treatment of choice, regardless of radiographic stage of the disease.

## 8.3 Calcaneal Lengthening Osteotomy

Instead of a lateral displacement calcaneal osteotomy, Ahmed et al. (Egypt, 2019) performed a calcaneal lengthening osteotomy in 13 feet of 7 adolescents, 5 girls and 2 boys, aged 14–17 (mean, 15.6 ± 0.98) years (Ahmed et al. 2019). Their BMI averaged 28.9 ± 2.89 (range, 26.2–34.4) kg/m$^2$.

Clinically, position of the hindfoot was neutral in 7 and mild valgus in 6 feet. Subtalar motion was painful with some restriction in all patients. In their first illustration, the left heel is said to be 'paradoxically neutral'. It looks in slight valgus with possible too many toes sign. Peekaboo sign may be positive on the right side.

Radiographically, all feet had a comma-shaped navicular with compression of its lateral portion, relative hypertrophy of the second metatarsal and an index minus metatarsal formula. On dorsoplantar radiographs, the authors measured the talo-first metatarsal and Kite's angles. On lateral radiographs, they assessed calcaneal pitch, Méary's and talo-calcaneal angles. All feet were at Stage IV according to Maceira's gradings.

In the consent process, parents were warned that osteotomy may not work, in which case arthrodesis might be required. Calcaneal lengthening was performed between the anterior and middle facets as described by Mosca (1995). Prior to distraction, the talonavicular and calcaneocuboid joints were stabilized with K-wires to prevent subluxation. The osteotomy was held open with a trapezoidal bicortical autogenous iliac crest bone graft and fixed with a K-wire.

Mean dorsoplantar talo-first metatarsal angles improved from 39.8° (range, 35–46°) preoperatively to 5.9° (range, 4–9°) postoperatively. Four feet had mild residual forefoot abduction. Mean calcaneal pitch angles increased from 7.5° preoperatively to 17.8° postoperatively. None of the patients required conversion to arthrodesis at a mean of 37.8 ± 11.83 (range, 24–64) months.

The authors pointed out that Maceira's study included patients as young as 13 years old. They rightly highlighted the lack of another series of adolescent patients with Müller-Weiss disease (MWD), which could be due to under-recognition or a low index of suspicion. They remarked that pes planus is an early feature in adolescent

MWD, while it is a later feature in more advanced or longstanding MWD. The medial prominence is formed by the navicular tuberosity in adolescent MWD, and not by the talar head as in progressive collapsing foot deformity (PCFD). Furthermore, considering that the feet were flat, the heels were not in excessive valgus, as in classic PCFD. The authors hence used the term '*paradoxically neutral*' to describe the neutral or mild valgus heel offset found in association with flatfoot deformity in adolescent MWD.

They also realized that the neutral heel position in 7 and mild valgus in the other 6 did not tally with Maceira's concept of heel varus as a hallmark deformity of MWD. They quoted other studies, which had also noted variable position of the heel in MWD, ranging from varus to neutral to valgus.

Ahmed et al. concluded that their calcaneal lengthening technique corrects flatfoot deformity and relieves pain while preserving joint motion. Theoretically, it should also relieve pressure off the lateral part of the navicular. Should osteoarthritis develop in future, it would be easier to perform arthrodesis of the realigned joints.

The first reaction to this rare approach of lengthening the lateral column is that it sounds at complete variance with contemporary opinion, especially the dogma of heel varus as a prerequisite for the diagnosis of Müller-Weiss disease. Indeed, published in the same issue of the journal follows a letter from Myerson to the authors disagreeing with their premise, hypothesis and conclusions (Myerson 2019). Myerson argues that the disease process always includes varus deformity at the hindfoot and subtalar joint, plus a flatfoot in more advanced Stages IV and V. The foot is rarely flexible in MWD, except perhaps to some extent in very early cases. Subtalar joint varus, Myerson maintains, must be corrected regardless of whatever else is done to the remainder of the foot. Since the deformities in Müller-Weiss disease are hindfoot varus and medial subluxation of the navicular off the talar head, it is impossible to correct deformity in MWD by lateral column lengthening, a procedure designed to adduct the midfoot and medially rotate the navicular for improving coverage of the under-covered talar head in flexible PCFD. In fact, since the navicular (and its tuberosity) always extrude medially in MWD, lateral column lengthening will only worsen this deformity and accentuate the medial foot prominence formed by the navicular tuberosity.

Myerson accepts that the navicular in Fig. 2 of Ahmed et al. is comma-shaped. However, *although he does not state his diagnosis,* he points out the radiographic features are not typical of MWD, because the heel and subtalar joint are not in varus like they should be *as also stated by all authors*. While the arch has improved following surgery, there remains a residual hindfoot valgus, which again is not consistent with the hallmark deformity of heel varus in MWD.

Myerson points out that, although reported in childhood, it would be extremely rare to have a cohort of children with MWD, all with early flexible deformity yet with flatfoot. Presence of the latter denotes advanced Stage IV or V disease, which would again be very rare in children. As the hindfoot was not in varus, he concludes the diagnosis of MWD in all of Ahmed's patients to be incorrect, adding that younger patients with MWD tend to have low BMI rather than raised BMI. He also disagrees that Müller-Weiss disease is a rare condition. He questions usage of a lateral column lengthening procedure, which would only worsen the medial prominence of the navicular tuberosity.

Ahmed, Kandil and Tabl anticipated the conflict that would arise from their unorthodox approach (Ahmed et al. 2019). In reply to Myerson's letter, the authors draw attention to the various other controversies surrounding aetiology, pathophysiology, natural history and treatment of the condition. They agree with Myerson regarding the rarity of Müller-Weiss disease in children. However, they rightly point out that Monteagudo and Maceira, other co-authors of Myerson, had stated that Müller-Weiss disease almost always starts in childhood, as in the *epidemic* and *non-epidemic* groups, and is suffered in adulthood. The adolescent feet in Ahmed's series were at Maceira Stage IV. Ahmed et al. commented that, as postulated by Maceira and Rochera, all 5 stages may develop progressively in infancy, when the navicular is still largely cartilaginous. Once ossification over, deformity does not progress, but the morphological changes remain. Maceira had also acknowledged that their classification was descriptive and had no prognostic value.

The authors go further disagreeing with Myerson on the concept of 'pes planovarus' deformity as a hallmark deformity of Müller-Weiss disease for the following reasons. Firstly, the term coined by Maceira does not apply to Stages I, II and III of the disease, as the medial arch only sags in Stages IV and V according to Maceira's own description of his classification. Secondly, *not all authors* have stated that the heel varus is a hallmark of the disease. In fact, other authors have also noted that the heel is not always in varus, with hindfoot position having been reported in neutral and valgus as well as varus. Hence, Ahmed et al. instead consider the comma-shaped navicular, resulting from compression of its lateral avascular sclerotic portion, as the hallmark deformity in Müller-Weiss disease regardless of heel position, and not heel varus.

In addition, they quote other studies that had also reported a raised BMI in patients with Müller-Weiss disease. They argue that the feet must have been flexible, as evidenced by clinical and radiographic correction following lateral column lengthening. Very few studies have actually studied movement at the subtalar joint in Müller-Weiss disease, some reporting reduced movements and others normal range of motion. During the preoperative planning, they had taken into consideration the possibility of worsening the medial talonavicular subluxation. Therefore, at surgery, K-wires were inserted across the talonavicular joint prior to distraction to pre-empt the complication that Myerson referred to. And this complication hence did not arise clinically or radiologically as evidenced by the postoperative radiographs.

Ahmed et al. accept that Müller-Weiss disease may not be a rarity, having noted its incidental presence in many trauma cases. They were referring to the rarity, among a whole spectrum of MWD, of their selected adolescent cases, where lateral column lengthening seems appropriate. They are not proposing that lateral column lengthening be applied to all cases of Müller-Weiss disease. Instead, conservative or operative treatment should be customized to the individual cases, be it osteotomy, calcaneal lengthening or arthrodesis.

## Concluding Remarks

Lateral displacement calcaneal osteotomy has been recommended as sole method of surgical treatment on the premise of obligatory heel varus as a hallmark deformity of Müller-Weiss disease. It works by redistributing load away from the diseased hyaline cartilage of the lateral navicular towards the healthy cartilage of the medial part of the navicular. Its proponents advocate it is worth trying, as arthrodesis can still be performed in future if required and will be easier done with a realigned calcaneum. However, it has also been shown by a study using hindfoot alignment radiographs that only 33% of heels were in varus. Caution is hence advised to ensure the heel is actually in varus before embarking along this line of approach, obtaining hindfoot alignment radiographs if necessary to confirm actual hindfoot orientation.

Instead of a lateral calcaneal slide, Egyptian surgeons report performing lateral calcaneal lengthening instead in early-onset disease. These adolescent feet appear to have a reverse Müller-Weiss pattern with markedly overlong second metatarsal and midfoot abduction. This would explain why lateral column lengthening works in these feet by simultaneous correcting midfoot abduction and restoring medial arch height. Geographical differences may exist which merit further investigations.

## References


Ahmed AA, Kandil MI, Tabl EA. Response to "Letter regarding: preliminary outcomes of calcaneal lengthening in adolescent flatfoot in Müller-Weiss disease." Foot Ankle Int. 2019;40(7):809–10. https://doi.org/10.1177/1071100719849430.

Ahmed AA, Kandil MI, Tabl EA. Preliminary outcomes of calcaneal lengthening in adolescent flatfoot in Müller-Weiss disease. Foot Ankle Int. 2019;40(7):803–7. https://doi.org/10.1177/1071100719833928

Avila A, Li S, Myerson M, Maceira E, Monteagudo M. The use of isolated calcaneus osteotomy in the treatment of Müller-Weiss disease. Foot Ankle Surg. 2016;22(2):83. https://doi.org/10.1016/j.fas.2016.05.209.

Fernández de Retana P, Maceira E, Fernández-Valencia JA, Suso S. Arthrodesis of the talonavicular-cuneiform joints in Müller-Weiss disease. Foot Ankle Clin. 2004;9(1):65–72. https://doi.org/10.1016/S1083-7515(03)00175-X

Fontaine R, Warter P, de Lange CH. La scaphoïdite tarsienne de l'adulte (maladie de Müller-Weiss). The adult tarsal scaphoiditis (Müller-Weiss disease) (In French). J Radiol Électrol. 1948;29(9–10):540–1.

Hetsroni I, Nyska M, Ayalon M. Plantar pressure distribution in patients with Müller-Weiss disease. Foot Ankle Int. 2007;28(2):237–41. https://doi.org/10.3113/FAI.2007.0237.

Janositz G, Sisák K, Tóth K. Percutaneous decompression for the treatment of Mueller-Weiss syndrome. Knee Surg Sports Traumatol Arthrosc. 2011;19:688–90. https://doi.org/10.1007/s00167-010-1305-z.

Li S, Myerson MS, Monteagudo M, Maceira E. The use of calcaneus osteotomy for treatment of symptomatic Muller Weiss disease. Foot & Ankle Orthop. 2016;1(1). https://doi.org/10.1177/2473011416S00104

Li S-Y, Myerson MS, Monteagudo M, Maceira E. Efficacy of calcaneus osteotomy for treatment of symptomatic Müller-Weiss disease. Foot Ankle Int. 2017;38(3):261–9. https://doi.org/10.1177/1071100716677741.

Lui TH. Arthroscopic triple arthrodesis in patients with Müller Weiss disease. Foot Ankle Surg. 2009;15(3):119–22. https://doi.org/10.1016/j.fas.2008.08.010.
Maceira E, Rochera R. Müller-Weiss disease: clinical and biomechanical features. Foot Ankle Clin. 2004;9(1):105–25. https://doi.org/10.1016/S1083-7515(03)00153-0.
Monteagudo M, Maceira. Management of Müller-Weiss disease. Foot Ankle Clin. 2019;24(1):89–105. https://doi.org/10.1016/j.fcl.2018.09.006
Mosca VS. Calcaneal lengthening for valgus deformity of the hindfoot. Results in children who had severe, symptomatic flatfoot and skewfoot. J Bone Joint Surg Am. 1995;77(4):500–12. https://doi.org/10.2106/00004623-199504000-00002
Myerson MS. Letter regarding: Preliminary outcomes of calcaneal lengthening in adolescent flatfoot in Müller-Weiss disease. Foot Ankle Int. 2019;40(7):808. https://doi.org/10.1177/1071100719849425.

# Chapter 9
# The Case for "Save as Many Joints as Possible"—The "SamJap" Approach

**Abstract** Although early researchers had cautioned against isolated talonavicular arthrodesis in Müller-Weiss disease, there is a trend reversal towards preserving the naviculocuneiform (NC), calcaneocuboid and subtalar joints wherever possible. Some centers perform in-situ talonavicular or triple arthrodesis without attempt at reducing medial talonavicular subluxation. Others effect reduction utilizing a lateral tension band principle or a pin distractor to derotate the plantar and medially displaced navicular lateralwards and dorsalwards to its normal location, and perform isolated talonavicular arthrodesis leaving the NC joints untouched unless they are severely affected. An interesting albeit perhaps unconventional 4-joint arthrodesis consists of a standard triple plus tricortical iliac crest bone graft interposed between the talar head and lateral cuneiform bone. The non-diseased NC1 and NC2 are left untouched. Several authors have also noted disease, often asymptomatic, at NC3 with healthy NC1 and NC2 joints, and have proceeded to isolated talonavicular or triple arthrodesis leaving the NC joints out of the fusion mass.

**Keywords** Müller-Weiss disease · Talonavicular arthrodesis · Lateral tension band · Double medial arthrodesis · Calcaneocuboid joint · 4-joint arthrodesis

## Introduction

Should the naviculocuneiform, subtalar and calcaneocuboid joints be preserved in the surgery for Müller-Weiss disease? So the debate goes.

Where achievable, Foot and Ankle Surgeons will typically opt for joint-preserving surgery instead of joint-sacrificing surgery, as discussed in the previous chapter. The "SamJap" perspective (Save as many Joints as Possible) described in this chapter aims to preserve as much motion as possible. The next chapter deals with selective arthrodesis, according to the joints involved. There will necessarily be some overlap between the "SamJap" and selective approaches.

The next subsection on talonavicular arthrodesis lists the studies in chronological order. The investigators in these articles chose to perform talonavicular arthrodesis alone based on the presumed absence of disease at the subtalar, calcaneocuboid and

© The Author(s), under exclusive license to Springer Nature Switzerland AG 2024

J. Wong-Chung, *Comprehensive Guide to Müller-Weiss Disease*,
https://doi.org/10.1007/978-3-031-66644-5_9

naviculocuneiform joints. However, other centres may well have performed different types of extended perinavicular arthrodesis for the examples shown. Hence, in these studies about to be discussed, the limits of talonavicular arthrodesis may have been stretched, and perhaps rightly so. Therefore, this author has elected to include them in this rather than in the next chapter on selective arthrodesis.

## 9.1 Isolated Talonavicular Arthrodesis

Fernández de Retana et al. (Spain, 2004) had warned against isolated talonavicular arthrodesis, because it carried a high rate of non-union and did not address disease at the naviculocuneiform joints (Fernández de Retana et al. 2004). Despite this initial cautionary note, various authors still limit arthrodesis to the talonavicular joint only, preserving the subtalar, calcaneocuboid and naviculocuneiform joints.

### *9.1.1 Isolated Talonavicular Arthrodesis Using a Lateral Tension Band Principle*

So as not to 'sacrifice' hindfoot mobility further, Fornaciari et al. (Switzerland, 2014) described their technique for performing isolated talonavicular arthrodesis using a lateral tension band principle in 10 feet of 8 women and 2 men with a mean age of 63 (range, 34–83) years old (Fornaciari et al. 2014). Three feet were at Maceira Stage III and 7 at Stage IV disease. According to the authors, excessive compression of the lateral part of the navicular between the talar head and the second metatarsal produced a "clamp-like" mechanism impairing its vascularity. Although hindfoot varus is a keyword, there is no further mention of hindfoot alignment throughout the whole article.

Surgery was performed through two separate incisions. After first exposing the talonavicular joint via a medial approach, a Hintermann distractor was used to distract the joint and prepare its surfaces. Maximum distraction of the medial joint space did not prove sufficient to reduce medial displacement of the navicular. A second dorsolateral incision was made to excise the fragmented lateral portion of the navicular and complete the joint preparation.

While maintaining maximum distraction at the medial talonavicular joint, the forefoot was maximally abducted. Fixation was initiated with a Uni-CP compression plate (Integra LifeSciences, Plainsboro, NJ) placed dorsolaterally. The first screw was inserted through the plate into the talar head. A second screw was next inserted into the dorsolateral part of the navicular, which was typically sclerotic. Tightening of this second screw pulled the navicular laterally. The remaining two other screws were inserted through the Uni-CP plate. Further reduction of medial talonavicular subluxation was achieved by spreading open the diamond-shaped bridge of the Uni-CP plate. Theoretically, the resulting stable lateral hinge construct allowed the tension effect of the tibialis posterior tendon to create compression at the arthrodesis site. To produce a lateral tension band, Hintermann hinted that the Uni-CP plate should be placed dorsolaterally and not laterally. Failure to do so resulted in implant failure in one patient, necessitating supplemental screw fixation.

Distraction was finally released on the medial side and stable fixation completed with two headless 5.5 mm Qwix compression screws (Integra LifeSciences, Plainsboro, NJ) across the medial aspect of the talonavicular joint (Fig. 9.1).

Except for the one foot that required additional screw fixation due to implant failure, all went on to solid fusion with improvement of AOFAS ankle-hindfoot score from 33 preoperatively to 88.3 postoperatively. In conclusion, the authors recommended talonavicular arthrodesis for disease limited to the talonavicular joint only, and not extending to either the subtalar or naviculocuneiform articulations. In 5 patients, SPECT-CT was said to have confirmed absence of activity in the other perinavicular joints.

However, their second and third illustrations depict an example of late-onset Group 3B Maceira Stage V disease involving the talonavicular more than the naviculocuneiform joint with fracture, dorsolateral extrusion of the lateral navicular fragment and formation of a talocuneiform articulation. Yet, cases are said not to have included those with involvement of the naviculocuneiform and subtalar joints. This author therefore included the study of Fornaciari et al. in this section, as the latter elected to perform isolated talonavicular fusion for these patients, whereas other surgeons may have preferred a talonaviculocuneiform arthrodesis with interpositional tricortical iliac crest bone graft instead.

### *9.1.2 Talonavicular Arthrodesis* In-Situ

Lu et al. (Taiwan, 2014) performed isolated talonavicular arthrodesis on 13 patients, 2 men and 11 women, aged 29–79 (mean, 55.6) years old (Lu et al. 2014). Two were at Maceira Stage III and 11 at Stage IV disease. The authors stated their preference for preserving the calcaneocuboid and subtalar joints, which were deemed relatively healthy 'with no obvious arthritic changes' in all their 13 cases.

Initially, they utilized a medial approach, which they found did not grant adequate access to the lateral part of the navicular. They subsequently changed to a dorsomedial approach that allowed excision of avascular bone fragments and better joint preparation. Fixation methods varied from staples to 6.5 mm headed cancellous lag screws and cannulated headless 4.3 mm compression screws.

Union rate was 76.9% with 3 nonunions, one of which was asymptomatic. In another nonunion, the dorsally extruded lateral navicular fragment that was previously left behind at index surgery, was removed along with medially situated metalwork. At surgery, partial union was noted at the medial and plantar aspect of the

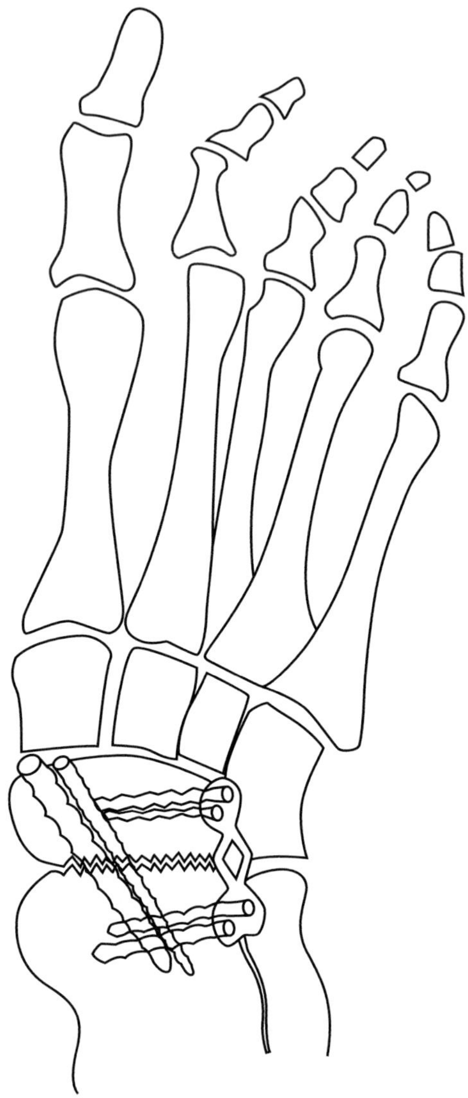

**Fig. 9.1** Schematic representation of the lateral band principle for talonavicular arthrodesis according to Fornaciari et al. Serrated edges denote the prepared joint surfaces. A 4-hole Uni-CP plate provides the lateral tension band. Two Qwix screws apply compression at the medial aspect of the talonavicular joint

talonavicular joint. The third foot with nonunion was revised to a Chopart arthrodesis and stabilized with staples.

Postoperatively, 8 feet developed arthritic changes in adjoining joints; 7 at the calcaneocuboid, 4 at both subtalar and calcaneocuboid, and 1 at the naviculo-cuneiform articulation. These degenerative changes did not affect outcomes, except in the same patient who underwent revision surgery to Chopart arthrodesis.

From their interpretation of the literature, core decompression has been performed in Stage I and excision of the lateral navicular fragment in Stage II disease. Based on their experience, they recommended isolated talonavicular arthrodesis for Stages III and IV but not for Stage V disease, where they considered triple, double or talonaviculocuneiform arthrodesis with abundant bone graft to be more appropriate.

Their first illustration depicts a Group 3B Maceira Stage V disease with dorsal extrusion of the lateral navicular fragment and direct articulation of the talar head with the lateral cuneiform bone. Talonavicular arthrodesis was performed and fixed *in-situ* with 2 staples. The dorsally extruded navicular fragment was left in place. There remained 35° of residual midfoot abduction.

Again, the works of Lu et al. are listed in this section, because of the authors' stated preference for conservation of the subtalar and calcaneocuboid joints. However, in the examples shown in their first and fifth illustrations, the naviculocuneiform joint is also involved as a result of dorsal extrusion of the lateral navicular fragment and formation of a talocuneiform articulation. Other centres may well have opted to treat these cases differently, performing a talonaviculocuneiform arthrodesis with interpositional tricortical iliac crest bone graft instead of talonavicular arthrodesis alone.

### 9.1.3 Talonavicular Arthrodesis in a Heterogenous Group

Harnroongroj and Chuckpaiwong (Thailand, 2018) acknowledged the controversy surrounding extension of arthrodesis to the naviculocuneiform articulations (Harnroongroj and Chuckpaiwong 2018). They remarked that all the different techniques in the literature appeared to yield uniformly good results. They reported the results of isolated talonavicular arthrodesis in 16 feet of 14 women and 2 men aged 47–70 years old, with normal calcaneocuboid and subtalar joints. All were at Maceira Stage III or above. *Patients younger than 18 years old were excluded.*

Surgery was carried out through a dorsomedial incision. Fixation was secured with two 3.5 mm cortical lag screws in 12, supplemented with a dorsal locking plate in the other 4 feet.

All 16 feet united within a median time of 2 months, although there were 3 delayed unions as defined by having taken over 3 months to heal. Significant improvement occurred in visual analogue scores (VAS) and Foot and Ankle scores ($p < 0.05$). While calcaneal pitch increased significantly, improvement in midfoot abduction and lateral Méary's angle did not reach statistical significance.

Two of their patients developed radiological osteoarthrosis at the naviculocuneiform joints at 12 and 18 months post index surgery, but were not symptomatic. Degeneration recorded preoperatively at the naviculocuneiform joint in 6 feet did not progress after surgery. Interestingly, they commented on the pattern of osteoarthritis in both feet that developed arthritis postoperatively and the 6 feet that had arthritis preoperatively at the naviculocuneiform joints. In all 8 feet, degenerative changes involved the lateral naviculocuneiform articulation only, the medial and middle naviculocuneiform joints having been spared.

Their illustrations reflect a non-homogenous mixture of cases. Thus, the feet shown in their first and seventh illustrations correspond to late-onset Group 3B Maceira Stage V disease affecting the talonavicular more than the naviculocuneiform joints, with marked medial extrusion of the navicular and direct articulation of the talar head with the lateral cuneiform. Postoperative radiographs as shown in their third illustration demonstrate marked residual midfoot abduction and medial subluxation with a prominent navicular tuberosity. Depicted in their fourth and fifth illustrations are late-onset Group 3A disease affecting the talonavicular joint only with mild medial talonavicular subluxation.

### *9.1.4 Talonavicular Arthrodesis with Reduction of Medial Subluxation*

Even with severe medial displacement of the navicular, Yuan et al. (Shanghai, China, 2019) argued the case for isolated talonavicular arthrodesis (Yuan et al. 2019). Utilizing a pin distractor to rotate the navicular lateralwards, they achieved reduction of medial talonavicular subluxation even in advanced Stages IV and V disease. In 36 feet aged 32–80 (mean, 53.6) years, they were thus able to perform 33 isolated talonavicular and only 3 talonaviculocuneiform arthrodeses. According to Maceira's classification, 9 feet were at Stage II, 10 at Stage III, 9 at Stage IV and 8 at Stage V.

Through a dorsomedial incision placed lateral to the anterior tibial tendon, the talonavicular joint was exposed and spread open with a pin distractor. The joint surfaces were prepared and avascular bone fragments excised. External rotation of the talar head was corrected by rotating the pin distractor in the horizontal plane until the talonavicular joint was reduced. Next, rotating the distractor in the sagittal plane reduced plantarflexion of the talar head (Fig. 9.2A–D). Temporary fixation was obtained with a K-wire. Reduction was verified under image intensifier on both dorsoplantar and lateral views. Permanent fixation consisted of a lag screw and an H-shaped dorsal locking plate. Autologous calcaneal bone graft filled any defect greater than 5 mm.

Out of 36 feet, Yuan et al. reserved talonaviculocuneiform arthrodesis for just 3 that had associated advanced osteoarthritis at the naviculocuneiform joint. They *only included the medial naviculocuneiform joint* in the fusion, leaving the middle and lateral naviculocuneiform joints untouched. Fixation was obtained with a 6-hole dorsal plate.

Their first figure illustrates a case of late-onset Group 3B Maceira Stage V disease affecting the talonavicular more than the naviculocuneiform joint with fragmentation and dorsal extrusion of the lateral navicular fragment. On postoperative radiograph, the navicular hardly appears reduced and is still markedly subluxed medially. There also remains residual midfoot abduction. Yet, the authors recorded significant improvement of calcaneal pitch, lateral Méary's angles, dorsoplantar talo-first metatarsal angles, talonavicular coverage and Kite's angles. Except for delayed union

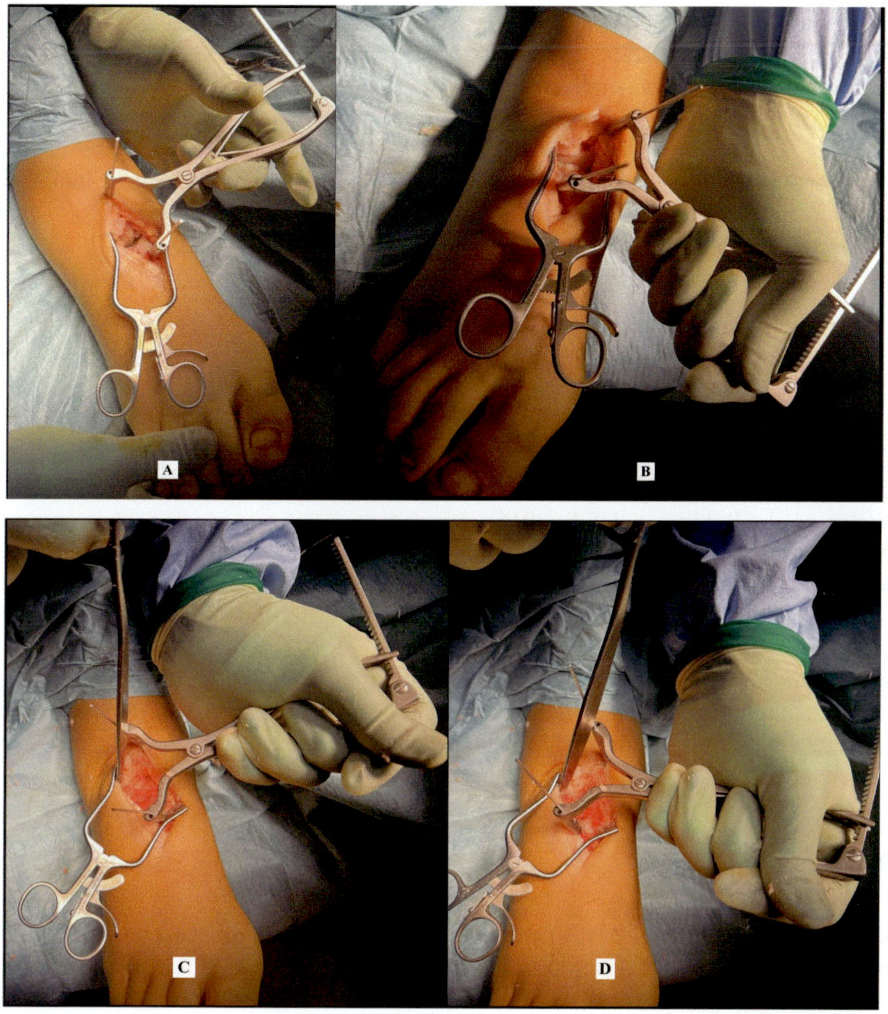


**Fig. 9.2** (A) Pin distractor in place across the unprepared talonavicular joint. Note medial subluxation of the navicular. (B) Rotating the pin distractor clockwise moves the talar head medialwards and reduces the navicular lateralwards. (C) and (D) Derotation of the navicular after joint preparation

in 1 patient, they reported a 97.2% union rate. AOFAS and VAS scores improved from 41.5 and 5.7 preoperatively to 85.3 and 0.9, respectively, after surgery ($p < 0.001$).

The authors believed that compression of the articular surfaces helped augment blood supply from the talus to the relatively less vascular navicular bone, thereby promoting chances of union. They realized that lengthening the medial column by derotating the talus in this fashion may generate increased joint reaction forces in both ankle and subtalar joints, which could explain why some of their patients continued to complain of pain postoperatively.

No additional gastrocnemius recession or calcaneal osteotomies were performed, as the calcanei were in normal position in all their patients. They further assert that, since the main problem is an imbalance between the talus and the navicular, repositioning of the talonavicular joint should automatically restore hindfoot alignment.

## 9.2 Talonavicular Arthrodesis and Lateral Displacement Calcaneal Osteotomy

### *9.2.1 Case Report*

Welck et al. (Baltimore, USA, 2016) reported on 3 patients, one of whom was a 53-year-old woman with Group 3A Stage IV disease (Welck et al. 2016). She was tender over the talonavicular joint. Although she was said to have subtle heel varus, hindfoot alignment view as depicted in their eighth illustration clearly showed valgus offset of the heel. Furthermore, a weight-bearing CT 3-D reconstruction image with its window level adjusted to show skin, confirmed the heel to be clinically in valgus, as per their ninth illustration. She underwent talonavicular arthrodesis combined with a lateralizing closing wedge calcaneal osteotomy.

### *9.2.2 Case Series*

Qu et al. (Xi'an, China, 2019) performed talonavicular arthrodesis combined with lateral displacement calcaneal osteotomy in 14 feet of 3 men and 11 women, aged 35–56 (average, 46.2) years (Qu et al. 2019). According to Maceira's gradings, 5 were at Stage III and 9 at Stage IV. Other than the talonavicular joint, none of the other perinavicular joints had arthritis according to the authors.

However, their illustration shows a case of Group 3B Maceira Stage III disease affecting both sides of the navicular, the talonavicular more than the naviculocuneiform joint with subchondral sclerosis and established osteophyte formation at the latter. In addition to a lateral displacement calcaneal osteotomy, arthrodesis of the talonavicular joint only was performed and stabilized with a headless lag screw medially and a compression staple laterally. The distal screw of the compression staple possibly infringes the lateral naviculocuneiform joint space.

Preoperative heel varus of $9.8 \pm 2.8°$ was corrected to $-2.5 \pm 2.7°$ postoperatively. On a Visual Analog Scale, pain decreased from $5.9 \pm 1.5$ preoperatively to $1.6 \pm 1.3$ postoperatively, while AOFAS ankle-hindfoot score improved from $58.8 \pm 17.6$ to $90.6 \pm 2.7$.

## 9.3 Triple Arthrodesis

Quoting Fernández de Retana, Maceira et al. (Spain, 2004) again, although triple arthrodesis provided better union rates, it does not address pathology at the naviculocuneiform joint (Fernández de Retana et al. 2004).

### *9.3.1 Arthroscopic Triple Arthrodesis*

While mostly performed by open method, Lui (Hong Kong, 2009) reported good results with in-situ arthroscopic triple arthrodesis in 6 women, aged 47–76 (mean, 67.75) years old (Lui 2009). No attempt was made to correct hindfoot alignment, as the patients only complained of joint pain and none about deformity or shoewear. According to Maceira's classification, 2 were at Stage IV and 4 at Stage V disease.

Preoperative radiographs demonstrated degenerative changes at the calcaneocuboid joint in 3 feet. No radiological abnormality was detected at the subtalar joints. Arthroscopy revealed degeneration at the talonavicular joint in all, at the subtalar in 1 and at the calcaneocuboid in 5 feet. Synovitis was present at the subtalar in 4 and calcaneocuboid joint in 2 feet. The author drew attention to the significant degenerative changes detected on arthroscopy at the calcaneocuboid articulations, but which were not visible on preoperative imaging.

All feet fused solidly within 16–22 weeks of surgery with improvement of AOFAS ankle-hindfoot score from 37.7 preoperatively to 81.5 at final follow-up. In one patient who complained of postoperative lateral foot pain when walking, pedobarography showed increased lateral sole pressure. Lui commented that she might have benefited from calcaneal dome osteotomy. Persistent mild degree of malalignment in all cases with a postoperative alignment score of 5 is explained by the fact that no deformity correction was attempted at surgery. One patient underwent calcaneal osteotomy for residual pain due to persistent varus.

Lui stated that his patients had no tenderness and no radiological evidence of arthritis at the naviculocuneiform joints. However, he illustrates a case of late-onset Group 3B Maceira Stage V involving the talonavicular more than the naviculocuneiform joint with fragmentation, dorsal extrusion of the lateral navicular fragment and formation of a talo-cuneiform articulation. The fixation lag screw appeared to have crossed from the lateral cuneiform distally into the talonavicular fusion mass proximally.

## 9.4 Triple or Talonavicular Arthrodesis

Wang et al. (Shanghai, China, 2012), believing they were the first to describe flatfoot in Müller-Weiss disease, reported on 6 patients, 5 women and 1 man with an average age of 54 years (Wang et al. 2012). Clinically, heel position was neutral in 3 and varus in 1. They performed isolated talonavicular arthrodesis augmented with autogenous iliac crest bone graft in 4 feet, without attempt at reducing medial subluxation even though all 4 had marked medial extrusion. The 4 feet represent late-onset Group 3B disease involving the talonavicular more than naviculocuneiform joints. One of the 4 feet was at Maceira Stage V with formation of a talo-cuneiform joint. The other 3 feet were at Stage III or IV.

In the other 2, they purportedly performed 2 triple arthrodesis. Their sixth case, representing a late-onset Group 3A Maceira Stage IV disease affecting the talonavicular joint only, was treated by a standard triple arthrodesis. Their third case looked more inflammatory than osteonecrotic in origin with concentric instead of eccentric arthritis. It underwent arthrodesis of the talonaviculocuneiform joint with a single longitudinal compression screw spanning the medial naviculocuneiform joint into the talonavicular joint. Distally, a transverse screw crosses the intercuneiform joints. The subtalar and calcaneocuboid joints were stabilized by screw fixation.

It is to be noted that Wang and three of his co-investigators are also named authors in the study from the same institution by Yuan et al. 7 years later (Yuan et al. 2019).

## 9.5 Modified Triple or 4-Joint Arthrodesis Versus Talonaviculocuneiform Arthrodesis

Zhang et al. (Suzhou, China, 2017) attempted to compare triple versus talonaviculocuneiform arthrodesis in 11 feet with Stage IV disease in 9 women and 1 man, aged 22–59 (mean, 48.1) years (Zhang et al. 2017). None had heel varus and the arch was high in only 1 foot.

Talonaviculocuneiform arthrodesis was performed in 6 feet via a dorsal longitudinal incision. Following joint preparation and excision of sclerotic bone, a bony bed was created, wider dorsally and narrower plantarwards. A tricortical iliac crest bone graft was inserted into the trough created and stabilized with dorsal plates and screws.

Triple arthrodesis also entailed creation of a bony bed, broader dorsally and narrower plantarward, into which a tricortical iliac crest bone graft was fitted in. An unspecified number of the 5 triples are not standard triple arthrodesis. Neither are they standard talonaviculocuneiform arthrodesis, but more like a hybrid between triple and talonaviculocuneiform arthrodesis. The authors actually refer to it as a "4-joint arthrodesis".

Their third illustration depicts a Group 3B Maceira Stage V, in which the talar head articulates directly with the lateral cuneiform bone. The standard triple joints were fused with no attempt at reducing medial talonavicular subluxation. In addition, a tricortical iliac crest bone graft was placed across the articulation between the talar head and the lateral cuneiform bone. Fixation was obtained with a dorsal locking plate spanning from the talar head, over the bone graft, and onto the lateral cuneiform (Fig. 9.3). The medial and middle naviculocuneiform joints were left untouched. This hybrid "4-joint arthrodesis" may deserve further evaluation especially in the late-onset Group 3B affecting the talonavicular more than the naviculocuneiform joint, where the medial naviculocuneiform joint (NC1) and all or part of NC2 often remain intact, as also highlighted by Wong-Chung et al., Harnroongroj and Chuckpaiwong (Harnroongroj et al. 2008; Wong-Chung et al. 2024).

Patient allocation was said to have been randomized to 5 open triple and 6 talonaviculocuneiform arthrodeses by a single senior surgeon, who also performed all the surgeries. Certain statements in the discussion call into question the randomization process. Most of the patients in the triple arthrodesis group had degenerative changes at the subtalar joint on CT scan. The senior surgeon proceeded to triple arthrodesis if arthritis was seen at the calcaneocuboid joint during surgery. Similarly, if the naviculocuneiform joint was involved, the triple was extended to include the naviculocuneiform joint. The authors concluded that they deemed it crucial to evaluate which joints are involved radiologically to guide selection of appropriate method of arthrodesis. They recommended triple arthrodesis for advanced disease, which tends to occur in relatively older patients in lesser need of hindfoot motion. In contrast, the patients who underwent talonaviculocuneiform arthrodesis were younger and had shorter union time.

The authors reported a 100% fusion rate. There was no significant difference in AOFAS scores between the 2 groups ($p = 0.1$). Average AOFAS ankle-hindfoot score improved from 30.2 to 79 in the open triple fusion group and from 33.2 to 86.2 in the talonaviculocuneiform group. The authors hence conclude that both modified open triple arthrodesis and talonaviculocuneiform arthrodesis are equally effective in the surgical treatment of Müller-Weiss disease.

## 9.6 Double Medial (Talonavicular + Subtalar) Arthrodesis

Wong-Chung et al. (2024) initially performed triple arthrodesis and subsequently changed to double medial arthrodesis to preserve the calcaneocuboid joint, retaining motion at the lateral column and avoiding lateral column pain that occurs after triple arthrodesis (Wong-Chung et al. 2024). (See also Chap. 10 on Selective arthrodesis).

**Concluding Remarks**

From a time of advocacy for talonaviculocuneiform arthrodesis, there is a revival to performing isolated talonavicular arthrodesis instead, preserving the calcaneocuboid, subtalar and especially the naviculocuneiform joints. Those who do usually strive for reduction of the medial talonavicular subluxation using a lateral tension band principle or a pin distractor to rotate the plantar and medially displaced navicular

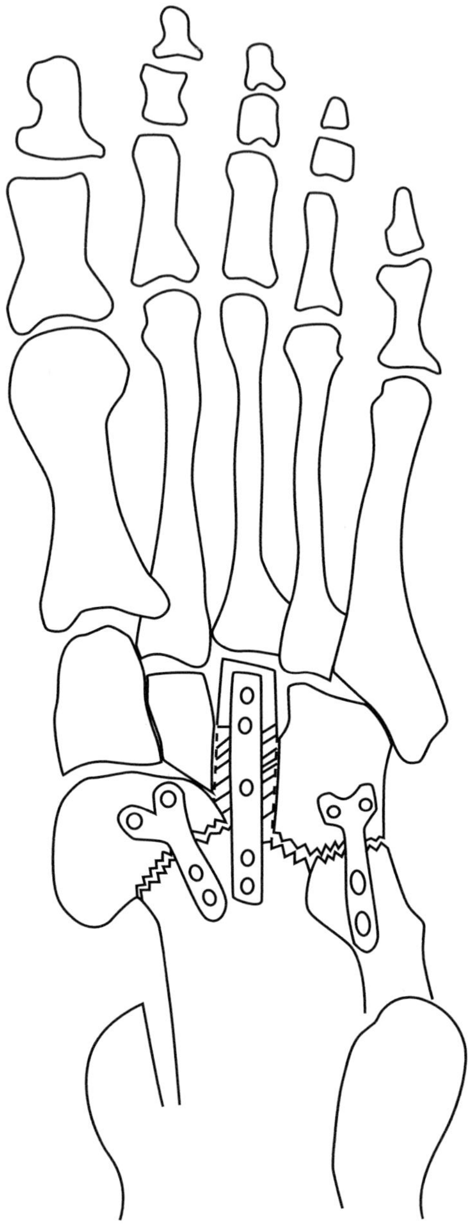

**Fig. 9.3** Schematic diagram of modified triple or 4-joint arthrodesis as described by Zhang et al. Joint preparation at the talonavicular, calcaneocuboid and lateral cuneiform denoted by serrated margins. Persistent medial extrusion of the navicular pole as talonavicular arthrodesis has been performed in situ and fixed with a dorsal Y-locking plate. Tricortical iliac crest bone graft (striped area) interposed between talar head and lateral cuneiform and stabilized with a bridging dorsal locking plate. Calcaneocuboid arthrodesis fixed with a Y-locking plate. Compression screw across the subtalar joint is not shown

laterally and dorsalward to its correct location. A few still perform in-situ talonavicular or triple arthrodesis. And others combine talonavicular arthrodesis with a lateral displacement calcaneal osteotomy to preserve the subtalar joint.

Some authors have noticed early but clinically asymptomatic involvement of the lateral naviculocuneiform joint. They have preserved the naviculocuneiform articulations and so far, have not noted progress of disease or need for further surgical intervention. An interesting offshoot from this concept is placement of an interpositional tricortical iliac crest bone graft between the talar head and the lateral cuneiform, leaving the non-diseased medial and intermediate naviculocuneiform joints intact. Combined with a triple arthrodesis, it has been termed a 4-joint arthrodesis. It may merit further investigation.

## References

Fernández de Retana P, Maceira E, Fernández-Valencia JA, Suso S. Arthrodesis of the talonavicular-cuneiform joints in Müller-Weiss disease. Foot Ankle Clin. 2004;9(1):65–72. https://doi.org/10.1016/S1083-7515(03)00175-X

Fornaciari P, Gilgen A, Zwicky L, Horn Lang T, Hintermann B. Isolated talonavicular fusion with tension band for Müller-Weiss syndrome. Foot Ankle Int. 2014;35(12):1316–22. https://doi.org/10.1177/1071100714548197.

Harnroongroj T, Chuckpaiwong B. Müller-Weiss disease: three- to eight-year follow-up outcomes of isolated talonavicular arthrodesis. J Foot Ankle Surg. 2018;57(5):1014–9. https://doi.org/10.1053/j.jfas.2018.01.008.

Lu CK, Fu YC, Cheng YM, Huang PJ. Isolated talonavicular arthrodesis for Müller-Weiss disease. Kaohsiung J Med Sci. 2014;30:471–6. https://doi.org/10.1016/j.kjms.2014.05.001.

Lui TH. Arthroscopic triple arthrodesis in patients with Müller Weiss disease. Foot Ankle Surg. 2009;15(3):119–22. https://doi.org/10.1016/j.fas.2008.08.010.

Qu F, Cai J, Liang X, Li Y, Lu J, Ji W, Zeng Q. Short-term effectiveness of talonavicular joint arthrodesis and calcaneus osteotomy for Müller-Weiss disease. [Zhongguo Xiu Fu Chong Jian Wai Ke Za Zhi] Chin J Reparative Reconstr Surg. 2019;33(2):166–9. https://doi.org/10.7507/1002-1892.201805036

Wang X, Ma X, Zhang C, Huang JZ, Jiang JY. Flatfoot in Müller-Weiss syndrome: a case series. J Med Case Rep. 2012;1(6):228. https://doi.org/10.1186/1752-1947-6-228.

Welck MJ, Kaplan J, Myerson MS. Müller-Weiss syndrome: radiological features and the role of weightbearing computed tomography scan. Foot Ankle Spec. 2016;9(3):245–51. https://doi.org/10.1177/1938640016630055.

Wong-Chung J, Blythe A, Lynch-Wong M, McKenna R, Wilson A, Stephens M. Outcomes of selective arthrodesis based on joints affected in 33 feet with Müller-Weiss disease. J Foot Ankle Surg. 2024;63(2):199–206. https://doi.org/10.1053/j.jfas.2023.11.001

Yuan C, Wang C, Zhang C, Huang J, Wang X, Ma X. Derotation of the talus and arthrodesis treatment of stages II-V Müller-Weiss disease: Midterm results of 36 cases. Foot Ankle Int. 2019;40(5):506–14. https://doi.org/10.1177/1071100719829457.

Zhang H, Li J, Qiao Y, Yu J, Cheng Y, Liu Y, Gao C, Li J. Open triple fusion versus TNC arthrodesis in the treatment of Mueller-Weiss disease. J Orthop Surg Res. 2017;12:13. https://doi.org/10.1186/s13018-017-0513-3.

# Chapter 10
# The Case for Selective Arthrodesis—Middle of the Road Stance

**Abstract** In between talonaviculocuneiform (TNC) arthrodesis and all joint-preserving surgery, there is a growing trend towards directing arthrodesis according to the joints involved in Müller-Weiss disease, as determined by clinical assessment and plain radiographs, and confirmed by either CT, MRI, SPECT-CT or diagnostic injections. None of the Wong Group 1 early-onset disease has required surgery so far. Fusion surgery in Group 2 Müller-Weissoid feet and Group 3A affecting the talonavicular joint only consisted of talonavicular or triple arthrodesis with a preference towards conserving the calcaneocuboid joint to preserve motion at the lateral column and performing a double medial arthrodesis instead. In both Groups 3B and 3C, TNC arthrodesis is performed supplemented with interpositional tricortical iliac crest bone graft in case of fracture or inadequate bone stock at the lateral navicular. In Group 3B, consideration can be given to performing isolated talonavicular arthrodesis if the naviculocuneiform joints are not symptomatic and medial talonavicular subluxation is adequately reduced.

**Keywords** Müller-Weiss disease · Selective arthrodesis · Talonavicular arthrodesis · Triple arthrodesis · Double medial arthrodesis · Talonaviculocuneiform arthrodesis

## Introduction

Somewhere in between talonaviculocuneiform arthrodesis fusing 2 rows comprising 4 joints and all-joints preserving surgery such as calcaneal osteotomy, others have recommended selective arthrodesis, according to which joints are affected.

To some extent, the studies in the previous chapter on 'SamJap' surgery would also carry some degree of selectivity. For example, performing an isolated talonavicular arthrodesis must perforce have necessitated the absence of gross disease at the subtalar, calcaneocuboid and naviculocuneiform joints. This chapter catalogues the works where the authors purposefully used specific imaging techniques such as CT, SPECT-CT or MRI to guide their choice of joints to arthrodese.

© The Author(s), under exclusive license to Springer Nature Switzerland AG 2024

J. Wong-Chung, *Comprehensive Guide to Müller-Weiss Disease*,
https://doi.org/10.1007/978-3-031-66644-5_10

## 10.1 CT

Cao and Miao (Zhejiang, China, 2018) based their decision-making on clinical signs and CT findings (Cao and Miao 2018). They carried out 12 talonavicular, 16 talonaviculocuneiform and 3 triple arthrodesis in 31 feet of 24 women and 4 men, aged 31 to 65 (average, 53.1) years. According to Maceira's grading, 3 feet were at Stage II, 15 at Stage III, 7 at Stage IV and 6 at Stage V. Solid union was achieved in all cases with excellent results in 8, good in 18 and fair in 5 feet. AOFAS score improved from 25.4 preoperatively to 80.3 postoperatively.

## 10.2 MRI

Having performed 9 talonaviculocuneiform arthrodesis for Maceira Stage III disease in 2012, Cao et al. (Chongqing, China, 2017) later recommended either talonavicular or talonaviculocuneiform arthrodesis according to which joints are involved, as determined by MRI scan (Cao et al. 2017). They performed isolated talonavicular arthrodesis in 16 feet of 2 men and 14 women, aged 35–62 (average, 50.3) years. None had evidence of disease at the subtalar or calcaneocuboid joints on MRI. Eleven of these had Stage III disease and were stabilized with two 4.0 mm cannulated headless screws. The other 5 with Stage IV disease had additional reverse V-shaped osteotomy through the talonavicular joint to restore the medial arch with supplemental autologous iliac crest bone graft.

Fourteen patients, 4 men and 10 women, aged 32–69 (average, 49.2) years, all of whom had Stage III disease and double row affection as determined on MRI, underwent talonaviculocuneiform arthrodesis with a reverse V-shaped osteotomy through the talonavicular joint. An autologous tricortical iliac crest bone graft was inserted into a rectangular trough fashioned on the dorsal aspect of the talonaviculocuneiform joint. It was stabilized with 2–3 cannulated 4.0 mm titanium screws. The foot was plantarflexed to restore medial column height and length. The illustrations demonstrate that the graft spans across the adjacent halves of the medial and middle naviculocuneiform joints and does not extend across the lateral naviculocuneiform joint.

All patients went on to solid fusion with decreased pain, improvement in mobility and quality of life. Mean AOFAS ankle-hindfoot score improved from 38.3 to 88.9 in the talonavicular group and from 40.1 to 90.1 in the talonaviculocuneiform group.

Cao et al. concluded with the recommendations of talonavicular arthrodesis when disease is localized to the talonavicular joint, and talonaviculocuneiform arthrodesis when disease involves both talonavicular and naviculocuneiform rows, for either Maceira Stage III or IV disease.

## 10.3 CT and MRI

As early as in 2004, Catonné et al. (France) had obtained CT in 14 feet and MRI scans in 5 to select which joints to fuse (Catonné et al. 2004). Accordingly, they performed 12 fusions: 1 triple, 2 Chopart, 7 isolated talonavicular, and 2 talonaviculocuneiform arthrodesis where the navicular was said to have been replaced with iliac crest bone graft. Long term results were good with pain relief and return to normal activity. Out of a total of 25 cases, the incidence appeared particularly high in black women aged 25–50 years old.

Liu et al. (Guangzhou, China, 2022) also utilized CT and MRI to decide on which joints to fuse in 12 feet of 11 women and 1 man, aged 49–73 (average, 58.3) years old, with Stage IV disease (Liu et al. 2022). CT was obtained in 8 and MRI scan in all 12. CT was useful in assessing deformity, remaining bone stock and arthritis, while MRI detected bone marrow oedema in the dorsolateral aspect of the navicular and effusion in adjacent joints. Overall, they found MRI more accurate than CT in evaluation of arthritis. All their patients had heel varus radiologically.

Eight of the 12 feet underwent isolated talonavicular arthrodesis. Three others were found to have calcaneocuboid arthritis also on CT and/or MRI and underwent arthrodesis of both talonavicular and calcaneocuboid joints. Medial subluxation of the navicular was reduced as much as possible. The talonavicular joint was stabilized with a fully threaded cannulated headless compression screw and a dorsal locking plate. The calcaneocuboid joint was fixed with two fully threaded cannulated screws.

Talonaviculocuneiform arthrodesis was performed in only 1 foot with fracture of the lateral navicular, marked medial talonavicular subluxation and dorsal extrusion of the lateral fragment and formation of a talocuneiform articulation. Degenerative changes were also present at the middle naviculocuneiform joint. This corresponds to a late-onset Group 3B Maceira Stage V disease, affecting the talonavicular more than the naviculocuneiform joint. Fixation consisted of (i) a fully threaded headless cannulated screw across an unreduced talonavicular joint medially, (ii) smaller fully threaded headless screw inserted retrogradely across the middle talonaviculocuneiform (TNC 2) and (iii) a dorsal locking plate with cancellous iliac crest bone chips across the third talonaviculocuneiform (TNC3) joint. *No fixation was used across the medial naviculocuneiform (NC1) articulation,* which appears not to have been prepared (Fig. 10.1).

Since the authors performed only one talonaviculocuneiform fusion, CT and MRI served mainly to detect changes at the calcaneocuboid joint. Their fourth illustration depicts marked degeneration at the talonavicular and calcaneocuboid joints on CT scan. It represents a Group 3B Maceira Stage V, with affection of the talonavicular more than the naviculocuneiform joint, marked medial extrusion and direct articulation of the talar head with the lateral cuneiform. It was treated by arthrodesis of an unreduced talonavicular and calcaneocuboid joints only.

One patient required revision for implant failure as a result of fully weight-bearing too soon after surgery. All feet eventually united with good patient satisfaction and improvement of AOFAS score from 62.5 to 95.3 ($p < 0.005$). Heel varus persisted

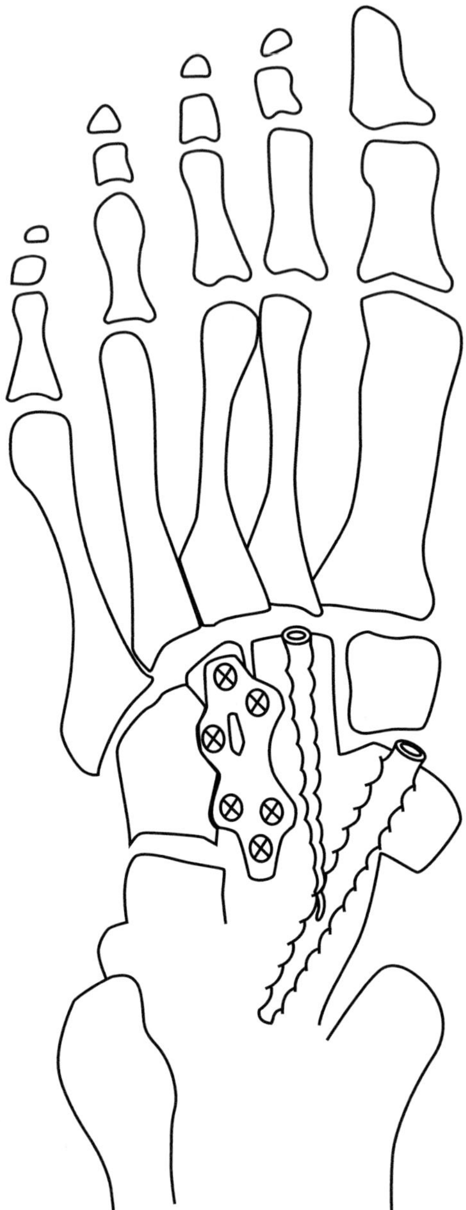

**Fig. 10.1** Schematic representation of arthrodesis and fixation as used by Liu et al. Fully threaded headless screw stabilizes an unreduced talonavicular joint medially. Smaller diameter fully threaded headless screw enters the middle cuneiform across the middle naviculocuneiform and talonavicular joint spaces into the talar head (TNC2). Dorsal locking plate and autologous cancellous iliac crest bone chips across TNC3. Unprepared medial naviculocuneiform joint

postoperatively in all patients. However, it had decreased radiologically from 7 ± 4.7° preoperatively to 4.9 ± 4.8° postoperatively. All the illustrations of postoperative radiographs demonstrate persistent postoperative medial extrusion of the navicular tuberosity.

## 10.4 SPECT-CT

Li and Zhang (Beijing, China, 2016) based their surgical decision-making on SPECT-CT findings in 5 feet of 4 women and 1 man, with a mean age of 52 years (Li and Zhang 2016). Although initial plain radiographs had suggested the presence of degeneration at the naviculocuneiform joints in 2 feet, SPECT-CT had subsequently revealed these joints to be normal. Surgery was hence limited to talonavicular fusion in 1 and triple arthrodesis in the other. Another foot, in which SPECT-CT had shown increased uptake at both talonavicular and naviculocuneiform joints, underwent talonaviculocuneiform arthrodesis. In one patient who continued to complain of pain following triple arthrodesis, SPECT-CT revealed arthritis with increased uptake at the naviculocuneiform joints. The fifth patient responded well to nonoperative treatment.

From the same centre 6 years later, Sun, Ebben, Li and co-authors (Beijing, China, 2022) reported the results of a larger prospective study on the use of SPECT-CT to guide treatment (Sun et al. 2022). They performed 3 talonavicular arthrodesis, 10 talonaviculocuneiform arthrodesis, 9 triple arthrodesis and 3 triple plus naviculocuneiform arthrodesis in 20 women and 4 men, with a mean age of 57.2 years. Maceira gradings were Stage II in 2 feet, Stage III in 8, Stage IV in 13 and Stage V in 2 feet.

Their third illustration depicts a case of Group 3B Maceira Stage V with the talar head articulating directly with the lateral cuneiform bone. It was treated by a triple plus naviculocuneiform arthrodesis. Postoperative plain radiographs demonstrate persistent marked medial talonavicular subluxation. Fixation was obtained with one retrograde screw across the medial talonaviculocuneiform articulation and a dorsal locking plate across the middle talonaviculocuneiform joint. There is no fixation and there does not appear to be interpositional bone graft across the lateral talonaviculocuneiform articulation. Three of the 12 feet did not unite and required additional surgery.

Al Khateeb et al. (Saudi Arabia, 2022) described a 55-year-old woman who gave more than one year's history of right foot pain (Al Khateeb et al. 2022). The hindfoot was said to be in valgus. Plain radiography and CT scan showed a Group 3B Stage V disease with dorsal extrusion of the lateral navicular fragment and resultant direct articulation of the talar head with the lateral cuneiform. Based on SPECT-CT findings, the authors proceeded to arthrodesis of the subtalar, talonaviculocuneiform and intercuneiform joints.

The extruded dorsolateral fragment, estimated at 40% of total navicular volume, was excised. The defect arising from its excision was filled with allograft bone. The subtalar arthrodesis was stabilized with two antegrade 5.5 mm cannulated compression screws. In contradiction with the authors' initial description of a valgus heel, heel varus was said to have been corrected at the subtalar joint just because the heel is meant to be always in varus in Müller-Weiss disease. For the talonaviculocuneiform fusion, a 2-hole Uni-CP compression staple spanned from the talar head into the medial cuneiform bone.

There remains persistent medial subluxation at the talonavicular joint. Outcome of surgery is not stated.

## 10.5 Surgery According to Joints Affected Including SPECT-CT for Guidance

In the retrospective study of a single surgeon's experience by Wong-Chung et al. (Northern Ireland, 2023), 33 of 64 feet failed to respond to an adequate period of nonoperative treatment and proceeded to arthrodesis (Wong-Chung et al. 2024). Surgery sites were initially guided by clinical location of pain and tenderness, plain radiography, CT and/or MRI. SPECT-CT supplanted the latter two modalities in the last 22 feet, when it became available at their institution in 2013. There were 10 men and 18 women, aged 26 to 78 (average, 59.2) years.

Isolated talonavicular arthrodesis was performed in 6 feet, in which disease was localized to the talonavicular joint. In 15 feet, disease extended to the subtalar joint. The first 8 of the 15 underwent triple arthrodesis. The author subsequently preferred double medial arthrodesis of the talonavicular and subtalar, leaving the calcaneocuboid joint alone in the other 7 to preserve some motion and obviate lateral column pain. In 4 feet with involvement of both talonavicular and naviculocuneiform joints but with adequate bone stock at the lateral navicular and without fracture, talonaviculocuneiform arthrodesis was carried out. In 2 of these 4, the subtalar joint was included as it was also symptomatic. In 6 feet with fracture and dorsal extrusion of the lateral navicular fragment resulting in direct articulation of the talar head with the lateral cuneiform (Maceira Stage V), talonaviculocuneiform arthrodesis was combined with an interpositional tricortical iliac crest bone graft (TICBG). A medial column plate with supplementary dorsal bridging locking plates conferred stable fixation of the talonaviculocuneiform fusions.

Of note, while the authors recognized the usefulness of SPECT-CT in guiding joint selection for arthrodesis, they also relied on physical examination actively seeking for tenderness at each perinavicular joint and combining the 2 methods to reach the final decision on which joints to fuse. For example, SPECT-CT not infrequently reveals mild isotope uptake at the lateral naviculocuneiform (NC3) joint and yet clinical examination demonstrates no tenderness at that joint. Surgery in these instances has been limited to isolated talonavicular, double medial or triple arthrodesis. Patients were informed of the risk of progression of degeneration at NC3, in which case fusion might need to be extended. So far, there has not been any need to do so nor has arthritis progressed at NC3, as also noted by Harnroongroj and Chuckpaiwong (2018). Similarly, the author has also performed isolated talonavicular and talonaviculocuneiform arthrodesis in the absence of pain and tenderness at the subtalar joint, despite early degeneration and increased radioisotope uptake at the anterior facet on SPECT-CT. Again, patients were warned that further extension may be required at a future stage and so far, none has required additional subtalar arthrodesis.

Union took place in 31 of 33 feet (94%) with significant reduction in pain interference and depression scores ($p < 0.001$) and concurrent increase in physical function ($p = 0.003$). Of the 2 non-unions, one had a fracture through the lateral navicular and the other marked sclerosis and avascularity of the lateral navicular. Based on their experience, the authors favour selective *à-la-carte* arthrodesis tailored to the individual case at hand instead of one-suits-all approach. In case of fracture or inadequate bone stock at the lateral navicular, they recommend talonaviculocuneiform arthrodesis with interpositional tricortical iliac crest bone graft. Adequacy of bone stock is best evaluated on medial oblique radiographs and CT scan.

## 10.6 Müller-Weiss Disease with Associated Asymmetric Varus Ankle Arthritis

Doyle, Napier and Wong-Chung (Northern Ireland, 2012) recounted their initial experience with 19 feet in 8 women and 4 men with a mean age of 57.9 years (Doyle et al. 2012). None gave a history of extreme environmental stress or poverty. Of 12 symptomatic feet, 7 proceeded to surgery. According to Maceira's gradings, 3 of 7 operated feet were at Stage III, 2 at Stage IV, and 1 each at Stages II and V. Surgery consisted of triple arthrodesis in 5. It was extended to include an arthritic naviculocuneiform joint as demonstrated on CT scan in 1 foot.

This 2012 study also comprised 2 patients with asymmetric varus ankle osteoarthritis, one of whom was a 68-year-old man with Müller-Weiss disease involving the talonavicular joint and heel varus. He had no pain and no tenderness at the talonavicular joint, which was hence left alone. He underwent total ankle replacement combined with lateral displacement calcaneal osteotomy.

The other, a 66-year-old farmer with involvement of the talonavicular and subtalar joints and concomitant end-stage asymmetric varus ankle osteoarthritis underwent pantalar arthrodesis. Seven years later, he underwent contralateral pantalar arthrodesis with preservation of the calcaneocuboid joint (Wong-Chung et al. 2024).

## 10.7 Surgery According to Wong Group

Wong-Chung et al. (Wong-Chung et al. 2023) analysed radiographs of 95 feet with Müller-Weiss disease and came up with 3 distinct groups according to (a) age of onset (b) previous evidence or absence of a radiologically normal navicular and (c) which joints were affected (See also Chap. 4 on Classification Systems).

Of the 95 feet, 37 underwent surgery. None of the feet in early-onset Group 1 (age, 9–29; mean, 22 years) had undergone surgery at final follow-up.

Eight of the 23 (35%) late-onset Group 2 Müller-Weissoid feet proceeded to surgery. These are the feet with previous evidence of a radiologically normal navicular 0.4–10.4 (median, 6.7) years earlier. Patient age at presentation ranged from 49 to 82 (median, 61) years. Degenerative changes predominated at the talonavicular joint, with early changes at the lateral naviculocuneiform (NC3) joint in 10 and moderate changes at NC2 and NC3 in 1 foot.

Late-onset Group 3 was subdivided according to the perinavicular joints involved. Only the talonavicular joint was affected in Group 3A. In Groups 3B and 3C, both sides of the navicular bone were involved. The talonavicular was more affected than the naviculocuneiform joint in Group 3B. The naviculocuneiform was more affected than the talonavicular joint in Group 3C. Eleven of the 16 Group 3A (69%), 12 of the 20 Group 3B (60%) and 6 of the 25 Group 3C feet (24%) required surgical intervention.

Surgery consisted of isolated talonavicular arthrodesis in the late-onset Group 2 Müller-Weissoid and Group 3A affecting the talonavicular joint only. If the subtalar joint was also symptomatic, they initially performed triple arthrodesis. They subsequently performed double medial arthrodesis of the subtalar and talonavicular joints, leaving the calcaneocuboid intact to preserve movement at the lateral column.

Talonaviculocuneiform arthrodesis was performed in both Groups 3B and 3C, where both talonavicular and naviculocuneiform joints are involved. In case of inadequate cancellous bone stock or fracture at the lateral navicular, the avascular sclerotic lateral fragment is excised and talonaviculocuneiform arthrodesis performed with an interpositional tricortical iliac crest bone graft held in place with bridging dorsal locking plates between the talar head and middle and lateral cuneiform bones. The authors prefer a medial column plate applied in compression mode across the talonaviculocuneiform joint (Table 4.1).

**Concluding Remarks**

In a continuing effort to preserve as many joints as possible, physicians resort to SPECT-CT or MRI ± diagnostic joint injections to guide selection of joints to be fused in Müller-Weiss disease.

In addition, the grouping system of Wong-Chung et al., which takes into account the joints involved, is useful for guiding surgery. None of the Wong Group 1 early-onset disease has required surgery yet. For Wong Group 2 Müller-Weissoid and Group 3A feet affecting the talonavicular joint only, surgery consists of isolated talonavicular or double medial arthrodesis if the subtalar joint is also symptomatic.

For Wong Groups 3B and 3C, surgery consists of talonaviculocuneiform arthrodesis supplemented with tricortical interpositional iliac crest bone graft in case of fracture or inadequate bone stock at the lateral navicular. In Group 3B, isolated talonavicular arthrodesis should be considered if the naviculocuneiform joints are asymptomatic and medial talonavicular subluxation is reduced (Table 4.1).

## References


Al Khateeb AM, Lozano RDPP, Al Khaldi M, Al SF. Which intervention may be most effective for Muller-Weiss disease. J Orthop Trauma Surg Rel Res. 2022. https://doi.org/10.37532/1897-2276.2022.17(3).71.

Cao HH, Lu WZ, Tang KL. Isolated talonavicular arthrodesis and talonavicular-cuneiform arthrodesis for the Müller-Weiss disease. J Orthop Surg Res. 2017;12(83):1–6. https://doi.org/10.1186/s13018-017-0581-4.

Cao L, Miao X. Selective arthrodesis for treatment of symptomatic Müller-Weiss disease. Foot Ankle Orthop. 2018;3(3). https://doi.org/10.1177/2473011418S00033

Catonné Y, Ribeyre D, Pascal-Mousselard H, Cognet JM, Delattre O, Poey C, Rouvillain JL. Aseptic osteonecrosis of the navicular bone: 25 cases. J Bone Joint Surg. 2004;86B(Suppl. 1):56.

Doyle T, Napier RJ, Wong-Chung J. Recognition and management of Müller-Weiss disease. Foot Ankle Int. 2012;33(4):275–81. https://doi.org/10.3113/FAI.2012.0275.

Harnroongroj T, Chuckpaiwong B. Müller-Weiss disease: three- to eight-year follow-up outcomes of isolated talonavicular arthrodesis. J Foot Ankle Surg. 2018;57(5):1014–9. https://doi.org/10.1053/j.jfas.2018.01.008.

Li S, Zhang J. The use of SPECT-CT in the diagnosis and surgical decision making for the treatment of Muller- Weiss disease: A prospective study. Foot Ankle Orthop. 2016;1(1). https://doi.org/10.1177/2473011416S00312

Liu W, Chen Y, Zeng G, Yang T, Ma M, Song W. Individual surgical treatment of stage IV Müller-Weiss disease according to CT/MRI examination: a retrospective study of 12 cases. Front Surg. 2022;17(9): 694597. https://doi.org/10.3389/fsurg.2022.694597.

Sun C, Ebben B, Li S, Zhu M, Myerson MS, Zhang M-Z. The use of SPECT-CT to define treatment for Müller-Weiss disease: a prospective radiographic and clinical study. Foot Ankle Orthop. 2022;7(4). https://doi.org/10.1177/2473011421S00958

Wong-Chung J, Walls A, Lynch-Wong M, Cassidy R, McKenna R, Wilson A, Stephens M. Towards understanding Müller-Weiss disease from an analysis of 95 feet. Foot Ankle Surg. 2023;29(5):401–11. https://doi.org/10.1016/j.fas.2023.05.004.

Wong-Chung J, Blythe A, Lynch-Wong M, McKenna R, Wilson A, Stephens M. Outcomes of selective arthrodesis based on joints affected in 33 feet with Müller-Weiss disease. J Foot Ankle Surg. 2024;63(2):199–206. https://doi.org/10.1053/j.jfas.2023.11.001

# Chapter 11
# Bone Graft Material in Müller-Weiss Disease

**Abstract** Various forms of autograft or allograft and bone substitutes have been used to replace all or almost all of the navicular in Müller-Weiss disease. They range from shaped femoral head and navicular allograft to autogenous free vascularized bone graft from the femoral condyle, iliac crest cancellous bone chips and calcium sulphate pellets.

**Keywords** Müller-Weiss disease · Allograft · Autograft · Biologics · Vascularized pedicle graft · Light bulb procedure

### Introduction

This chapter focuses on works that rely substantively on allograft or autograft to replace the entire or almost all of the navicular, and not just as an adjunct to supplement arthrodesis. It includes use of vascularized grafts, but does not include an interpositional tricortical iliac crest bone graft to replace the excised avascular lateral navicular fragment (See Chap. 7).

## 11.1 Femoral Head Allograft

Tan et al. (Netherlands, 2011) shaped a femoral head allograft to replace the *entire* navicular bone, supplementing it with autologous iliac crest cancellous bone chips, in a 51-year-old woman with Stage IV Müller-Weiss disease (Tan et al. 2011). Fifteen years earlier, she had excision of a neuroma of the deep peroneal nerve, a complication which had arisen following a previous ankle ligament reconstruction. She had remained pain-free since until she presented with spontaneous onset of the new symptoms. No mention is made of radiographic findings from around the time of the previous two surgeries.

Plain radiographs demonstrate established degenerative changes at the talonavicular and calcaneocuboid joints. Compression of the lateral navicular and medial

© The Author(s), under exclusive license to Springer Nature Switzerland AG 2024 
J. Wong-Chung, *Comprehensive Guide to Müller-Weiss Disease*,
https://doi.org/10.1007/978-3-031-66644-5_11

extrusion appear mild. The medial arch sags at the naviculocuneiform joints, which are mostly intact on plain radiographs and MRI. SPECT-CT shows marked radioisotope uptake at the talonavicular joint, and quiescent calcaneocuboid and naviculocuneiform joints. There may be a hint of irregularity of the articular surface at the cuneiform side of the lateral navicular on SPECT-CT, but there is no fragmentation. The second metatarsal is substantively longer than the first. The foregoing description fits in with a Group 3A Maceira Stage IV disease.

At surgery, the navicular was found to be 'fragile' with severe necrosis. It was completely excised and replaced with a 'new' navicular. Fixation was secured with a dorsal 8-hole AO T-plate with 3 screws engaging into the talar head proximally and 2 into the medial cuneiform distally. Metalwork was subsequently removed after sound bony union had occurred.

MRI and SPECT-CT images do not demonstrate necrosis of the entire bone with good signal intensity of the navicular bone marrow medially right up to its lateral third. A more limited operation such as talonavicular ± calcaneocuboid arthrodesis may well have sufficed.

## 11.2 Femoral Head and Navicular Allograft Strut

Lee et al. (Taiwan, 2022) reported midterm results of arthrodesis using a strut allograft in 20 feet of 4 men and 16 women, aged 19 to 80 (mean, 59.6 ± 15.6) years old (Lee et al. 2022). Average BMI was 25.9 ± 3.53 kg/m$^2$. Maceira stages were II in 4, III in 6, IV in 4 and V in 6 patients. The authors expressed concern at the lack of adequate structural support and mechanical stability with morselized bone graft, which could result in shortening or collapse of the medial column. They therefore used strut graft shaped from femoral head allograft in 18 and from navicular allograft in 2 cases. It was also applied at the subtalar and calcaneocuboid articulations as required. A single surgeon performed 9 triple arthrodesis, 7 double medial and 4 double medial with additional interpositional calcaneocuboid arthrodesis. Surgery was carried out via a medial with supplemental dorsolateral incision if needed.

Radiographic correction of calcaneal pitch, talonavicular coverage, dorsoplantar and lateral Méary's angles averaged at least 50% in feet at Maceira Stages II and III, and up to 80% in feet at Maceira Stages IV and V.

Postoperative radiographs are shown of a double medial arthrodesis performed for a Group 3B Maceira Stage V disease with formation of a talo-cuneiform articulation. Either there is persistent medial subluxation or talonavicular arthrodesis may have been performed in-situ and stabilized with a medial locking plate. The proximal inferior plate screw is broken and union looks incomplete. A shaped allograft appears to have been fixed to the lateral half of the talar head with 2 cannulated screws. No medial oblique view is provided. The naviculocuneiform joints have been left intact. It is therefore uncertain how the strut graft affixed onto the lateral part of the talar head articulates with the lateral cuneiform bone, when there is persistent medial displacement of the navicular.

Reported union rate was 100% with a union time of 4.0 ± 1.6 months. According to their Table 4, there was no implant failure either. However, the aforementioned radiographs had demonstrated broken hardware with incomplete talonavicular union. The same patient was said to have no discomfort or limitation of movements. Pain at the fourth and fifth tarsometatarsal joint respectively in 2 patients was thought not to be related to the surgery and responded to shoe modification.

The authors concluded that allograft was conducive to favourable bone healing while allowing fashioning of any size or shape of graft, obviating the need for harvesting autogenous bone and thereby avoiding donor site morbidity.

## 11.3 Autogenous Free Vascularized Bone Graft for Maceira Stage I Disease

Levinson et al. (Durham, NC, USA, 2013) reported on a case of a 25-year-old man, whose plain radiographs were normal and MRI showed signal intensity changes throughout the left navicular with maintenance of bone height and no associated fragmentation (Levinson et al. 2013). These findings would correspond to a Maceira Stage I disease.

After 2 years of failed nonoperative treatment, the authors chose to implant a free vascularized bone graft harvested from the medial femoral condyle along with its descending genicular vascular pedicle. The entire medullary cavity of the navicular bone was debrided, while preserving the endocortical shells of the proximal and distal articular surfaces. The vascularized bone graft was inserted into the cavity with end-to-side anastomosis of the genicular to the dorsalis pedis vessels.

At final follow-up of 18 months, the patient is doing well, has no pain and has regained normal function.

## 11.4 Autogenous Iliac Crest Cancellous Bone Chips

Two years earlier, Tosun et al. (Turkey, 2011) had described a similar technique in a 43-year-old man (Tosun et al. 2011; Nelson and Rivello 2012). Plain radiography showed diffuse increase in bone density throughout the right navicular. CT scan demonstrated sclerosis with cyst formation within the central and lateral third of the navicular and irregularity of its proximal articular surface but no gross bone loss or collapse. MRI scan revealed bone marrow oedema within the central and lateral third of the navicular, irregular cortical margins and a sclerotic line adjacent to the subchondral bone plate. Imaging features were deemed consistent with an osteonecrotic process. It may represent a Maceira Stage I disease.

Through a circular dorsomedial corticotomy, all the avascular intramedullary bone were removed using curettage and a high-speed burr until only the cortical shell remained. The void thus created was replaced with ipsilateral iliac crest cancellous bone chips.

Histopathological examination confirmed an osteonecrotic process with no evidence of infection or neoplasm. At 3 years' follow-up, the patient had made a full recovery with satisfactory incorporation of the bone graft without bone collapse or progression of degeneration.

## 11.5 Light Bulb Procedure

Chang et al. (Taiwan, 2019) performed a similar procedure in a 37-year-old woman who initially presented with an osteochondral lesion of the medial talar dome (OLT) and ipsilateral Stage I Müller-Weiss disease as diagnosed by low T1 and high T2 signal intensities throughout the navicular bone on MRI scan (Chang et al. 2019). After 3 months of failed nonoperative treatment, she underwent arthroscopic microfracture awl of the OLT and percutaneous decompression of the navicular. While ankle pain improved, midfoot pain persisted with an AOFAS midfoot score of 39. Repeat MRI at 6 months revealed persistent osteonecrosis and CT scan demonstrated sclerotic changes with loss of trabecular structure.

The authors performed a 'light bulb' procedure akin to that described by Rosenwasser et al. for avascular necrosis of the femoral head (Rosenwasser et al. 1994). Through a dorsal approach, a bone window was created in the navicular. All sclerotic necrotic bone was removed using a high-speed burr. Care was taken not to perforate cortical bone. Extent of débridement was verified by shining an arthroscopic light source at the medial aspect of the navicular. Before débridement, transillumination through sclerotic bone was weak. Following thorough debridement, the navicular transilluminated brightly. The resulting cavity was filled with calcium sulphate pellets (Osteoset®, Wright Medical, Memphis, TN) and the cortical window replaced.

Her symptoms resolved within 3 months. At 6 years' final follow-up, she remained asymptomatic with an AOFAS midfoot score of 97. MRI revealed remodeling of the navicular with small areas of low signal intensity on T1 sequences. Plain radiographs showed low-grade perinavicular degenerative changes with no bone collapse or deformity.

## 11.6 Medial Navicular Remnant Versus Autogenous Tricortical Iliac Crest Bone Graft to Replace Whole Navicular

Jones et al. (Brazil, 2022) questioned whether it is worthwhile keeping the navicular bone in the surgery of Müller-Weiss disease. (Alcântara et al. 2022) The authors came up with the idea of using the medial navicular remnant as interpositional bone graft, since this portion is usually viable. It has the same properties as iliac crest bone and would obviate the need for harvesting. They compared the results of surgery using an autogenous tricortical iliac crest bone graft versus use of the medial navicular remnant as interpositional bone graft to replace the entire navicular. The decision whether to use tricortical iliac crest bone graft or the medial navicular remnant rested with the individual surgeon.

The entire navicular was excised and replaced with a tricortical iliac crest bone graft in 6 feet (Group A). Talonaviculocuneiform arthrodesis was extended to include the subtalar and calcaneocuboid joints in 1 foot and the first tarsometatarsal joint in 2 feet. Fixation was obtained with plate and screws in 5 and K-wires only in 1.

In 6 other feet (Group B), the medial navicular remnant was used as interpositional bone graft. Surgery consisted of arthrodesis of the talonavicular joint only in 2, triple in 2, talonaviculocuneiform in 1, and triple and naviculocuneiform in 1. Fixation was obtained with screws in 4 and K-wires only in 2.

Age at time of surgery ranged from 23 to 56 (mean, 44) years. Each group had 4 feet at Stage III and 2 at Stage IV. Two feet from each group developed nonunion. Three of the 4 nonunions underwent successful revision surgery, while the fourth patient declined further surgery.

Presumably in the Group B feet, the medial half to two-thirds of the navicular bone were released and mobilized. It is not specified whether the medial navicular remnant was wide enough to span the entire space between the talar head and the three cuneiform bones. Nor do the authors state how they dealt with the insertion of the posterior tibial tendon. No illustration of a preoperative radiograph or postoperative fixation is provided. The authors acknowledged the retrospective nature of their study, the small sample and a high nonunion rate of 33%.

## 11.7 Vascularized Free Scapular Bone Graft

Toren et al. (Colorado, USA, 2013) reported on a 17-year-old man who injured his left foot while playing indoor lacrosse (Toren et al. 2013). He underwent primary open reduction and internal fixation for a presumed stress fracture through the lateral third of the navicular. Nine months later, the presumed fracture had still not united. Revision surgery consisted of hardware removal and application of demineralized bone matrix. Screw fixation, from medial to lateral, engaged into the cuboid for greater stability. CT scan obtained at 5 months after the second surgery demonstrated persistent nonunion, narrowing of the talonavicular joint space, cystic degeneration and sclerosis at the lateral navicular suggestive of avascular necrosis. Third surgery consisted of excision of the avascular lateral navicular fragment, talonaviculocuneiform and calcaneocuboid arthrodesis.

Repeat CT scan obtained 1 year later for increasing midfoot pain revealed 25% bony union across the talonavicular, 45% at the naviculocuneiform and 95% bony union across the calcaneocuboid joint. Lucency was present around several medial column screws, one of which had broken. With the collaboration of a microvascular surgeon, a free vascularized lateral scapular bone fragment with its circumflex scapular artery and vein was applied to the medial column. The 4-cm bone graft was secured in place with 2 medio-lateral screws. The vessels were anastomosed to the posterior tibial artery and vein. Solid bony union ensued at the 12-week mark.

Analysis of the early plain radiographs and CT scan shows obvious compression of the lateral part of a comma-shaped navicular with fracture at the level of the lateral intercuneiform joint, medial talonavicular subluxation with medial extrusion of the navicular pole, subchondral cyst formation, subchondral sclerosis and obliteration of the lateral talonavicular joint space. The appearances are consistent with an early-onset Müller-Weiss disease in a foot with marked overlength of the second metatarsal relative to the first—similar to the early-onset Group 1 disease as described by Wong-Chung et al. (2023).

This case illustrates underdiagnosis of the condition, which is often mistaken for a navicular stress fracture. Had the diagnosis of Müller-Weiss disease been considered at outset, surgical treatment would have consisted of talonaviculocuneiform arthrodesis with interpositional tricortical iliac crest bone graft. Instead, it took 4 surgeries to resolve the problem, when just one might have sufficed.

## 11.8 Local Vascularized Pedicle Bone Grafting

Fishman et al. (North Carolina, USA, 2012) performed local vascularized pedicle bone grafting for nonunion following trauma in 1 and stress fracture in 2 naviculars (Fishman et al. 2012). Their series also included 5 cases of osteonecrosis of the navicular, of which 2 had associated arthritis of the talonavicular joint. The article shows illustrations of the surgical technique but no example of pre or post-operative radiographs. However, they refer to Müller-Weiss disease as a cause of osteonecrosis. Perhaps, the 5 feet or at least the 2 feet with osteonecrosis and concomitant talonavicular arthritis might have had Müller-Weiss disease.

### Concluding Remarks

A variety of allograft, biologics, free or vascularized autograft have been used to replace all or most of the navicular or to enhance union. Choice of graft depends also on availability to the surgeon. For example, not all foot and ankle units have access to whole navicular allografts or a Plastic Surgery Service for vascularized pedicle grafts.

Interestingly, some procedures were performed for Maceira Stage I as first line of treatment. In another instance, the whole navicular was replaced with allograft whereas others might have opted for a simpler talonavicular ± calcaneocuboid arthrodesis.

Autograft, either in the form of cancellous bone chips or tricortical iliac crest bone graft, remains the ‘old reliable’, especially when dealing with unhealthy bone to start with. It can be supplemented with bone marrow aspirate concentrate.

# References

Chang SM, Chen PY, Tsai MS, Shee BW. Light bulb procedure for the treatment of tarsal navicular osteonecrosis after failed percutaneous decompression: a case report. J Foot Ankle Surg. 2019;58(1):187–91. https://doi.org/10.1053/j.jfas.2018.08.003.

de Alcântara Jones D, Belzarena AC, Costa MT, Ferreira RC. Arthrodesis in Müller-Weiss disease: is it worth keeping the navicular bone? J Foot and Ankle. 2022;16(3):248–252. https://doi.org/10.30795/jfootankle.2022.v16.1664

Fishman FG, Adams SB, Easley ME, Nunley JA. Vascularized pedicle bone grafting for nonunions of the tarsal navicular. Foot Ankle Int. 2012;33:734–9. https://doi.org/10.3113/FAI.2012.0734.

Lee TY, Wu CC, Yang KC, Yeh KT, Chen IH, Wang CC. Midterm outcomes of midfoot and hindfoot arthrodesis with strut allograft for Müller-Weiss disease. BMC Musculoskelet Disord. 2022;23:715. https://doi.org/10.1186/s12891-022-05629-7.

Levinson H, Miller KJ, Adams SB, Parekh S. Treatment of spontaneous osteonecrosis of the tarsal navicular with a free medial femoral condyle vascularized bone graft. A new approach to a managing a difficult problem. Foot Ankle Spec. 2013;7(4):332–337. https://doi.org/10.1177/1938640013514270

Nelson EW, Rivello G. A case of Müller-Weiss disease of the tarsal navicular. J Foot Ankle Surg. 2012;51(1):141; author reply 141. https://doi.org/10.1053/j.jfas.2011.10.023

Rosenwasser MP, Garino JP, Kiernan HA, Michelsen CB. Long term followup of thorough debridement and cancellous bone grafting of the femoral head for avascular necrosis. Clin Orthop Relat Res. 1994;306:17–27.

Tan A, Smulders YC, Zöphel OT. Use of remodeled femoral head allograft for tarsal reconstruction in the treatment of Müller-Weiss disease. J Foot Ankle Surg. 2011;50(6):721–6. https://doi.org/10.1053/j.jfas.2011.04.043.

Toren AJ, Hahn DB, Brown WC, Stone PA, Ng A. Vascularized scapular free bone graft after nonunion of a tarsal navicular stress fracture: a case report. J Foot Ankle Surg. 2013;52(2):221–6. https://doi.org/10.1053/j.jfas.2012.12.010.

Tosun B, Al F, Tosun A. Spontaneous osteonecrosis of the tarsal navicular in an adult: Mueller-Weiss syndrome. J Foot Ankle Surg. 2011;50(2):221–4. https://doi.org/10.1053/j.jfas.2010.10.019.

Wong-Chung J, Walls A, Lynch-Wong M, Cassidy R, McKenna R, Wilson A, Stephens M. Towards understanding Müller-Weiss disease from an analysis of 95 cases. Foot Ankle Surg. 2023;29(5):401–11. https://doi.org/10.1016/j.fas.2023.05.004.

# Chapter 12
# Treatment for Bipartite Navicular and Brailsford's Osteochondritis

**Abstract** Conditions labelled as bipartite navicular and severe forms of Brailsford's osteochondritis represent Maceira stage V of Müller-Weiss disease, whereby the lateral portion of the navicular has fragmented, the small lateral navicular fragment extruded dorsally, the larger medial fragment subluxed medially and the talar head articulating directly with the lateral cuneiform bone forming the talocuneiform articulation. Open reduction and internal fixation of the lateral navicular fragment to the parent bone has been attempted with mostly poor outcomes, as anticipated by Fernández de Retana et al. who warned that the lateral navicular fragment is far too small for bony union. Others have performed talonavicular arthrodesis and either excised the dorsally extruded lateral navicular fragment or fused it to the lateral cuneiform bone to supposedly preserve motion through the so-called crank-shaped arthrodesis.

**Keywords** Müller-Weiss disease · Bipartite navicular · Brailsford's osteochondritis · Internal fixation · Talonavicular arthrodesis · Crank-shaped arthrodesis

## Introduction

This Chapter relates instances of treatment for conditions diagnosed as bipartite navicular or Brailsford's osteochondritis. As discussed in Chap. 1, this author believes the more severe forms of bipartite navicular and Brailsford's osteochondritis actually represented Stage V Müller-Weiss disease on Maceira's classification, whereby the lateral navicular fragment displaced dorsally and laterally, while the medial fragment subluxed medially and the talar head ultimately articulated directly with the lateral ± middle cuneiform bones.

The term bipartite navicular pertains only to cases with splitting of the navicular, whatever the degree of separation of fragments but usually with wide fragment separation. The terms Brailsford's osteochondritis and Müller-Weiss disease include feet with and without fragmentation.

© The Author(s), under exclusive license to Springer Nature Switzerland AG 2024
J. Wong-Chung, *Comprehensive Guide to Müller-Weiss Disease*,
https://doi.org/10.1007/978-3-031-66644-5_12

## 12.1 Open Reduction and Internal Fixation for So-Called Bipartite Navicular

Yamaguchi et al. (Japan, (2016) reported their results with open reduction and internal fixation of so-called 'bipartite naviculars' in two 14-year-old adolescent male soccer players (Yamaguchi et al. 2016). In their own words, the fragmented "navicular appeared comma-shaped owing to the flattened lateral half of the bone" with dorsal displacement of the lateral fragment. CT scan revealed dorsolateral and plantar-medial fragments with sclerotic margins and marginal osteophytes. After failed nonoperative treatment, surgery was undertaken consisting of meticulous curettage of the bone ends with chisels and curettes. Autologous cancellous iliac crest bone graft was inserted into the bony defect. Fixation was obtained with a variable threaded screw and an autologous bone pin. Low intensity pulsed ultrasound was applied postoperatively to stimulate bone healing. CT scan at 3 months showed union and gradual return to sports was permitted. However, repeat CT scan at 8 months after surgery demonstrated separation of the bone fragments with established nonunion. At 3 years' follow-up, he still complained of pain.

Their second case exhibited similar radiographic findings. The dorsolateral fragment was superimposed upon the lateral cuneiform bone and osteophyte formation was present at the dorsal aspect of the middle cuneiform. A further fracture line was identified on CT scan in the middle of the dorsolateral fragment between the central and lateral third of the navicular. Its margins were not sclerotic and displayed bone marrow oedema on MRI. A diagnosis of bipartite navicular with stress fracture of the dorsolateral fragment was hence made. He underwent a similar procedure with autologous cancellous bone graft from the proximal tibia and fixation with 2 tapered variable threaded screws. As union appeared to be proceeding on repeat CT scan at 6 months postoperatively, the patient was allowed to resume sports. Again, further CT scanning at 10 months showed separation of the bone fragments with loosening of the screws and confirmed nonunion. Although arthritis had not progressed in either case at 2 to 3 years' follow-up, both feet remained painful with Japanese Society for Surgery of the Foot (JSSF) midfoot scales of 80 and 87 respectively.

The literature had not contained any previous report of surgical treatment for painful bipartite navicular in children. In view of their poor experience, Yamaguchi et al. counselled against internal fixation of the so-called bipartite navicular due to recurrence of separation of the bone fragments upon resumption of physical activity, even though union appeared to have occurred at some earlier stage.

Fernández de Retana et al. had warned that the lateral bone fragment may be too small for internal fixation in Müller-Weiss disease (Fernández de Retana et al. 2004). Yamaguchi et al. reached the same conclusion for presumed bipartite naviculars. Likewise, they recommended that talonaviculocuneiform or talonavicular arthrodesis should have been considered instead.

In contrast, Alomran et al. (Hamilton, Ontario, Canada, (2024) reported a favorable outcome with bony union at 3 months following screw fixation of a very small lateral navicular fragment and grafting with synthetic calcium phosphate (Alomran et al. 2024). They believed their 16-year-old male patient to be the youngest ever reported patient with Müller-Weiss disease. He gave a one-year's history of gradual onset of midfoot pain without recall of injury. He was treated with analgesia and immobilization in an Aircast Walker for 3 weeks. The authors believed his pain would not have settled down due to instability of the lateral fragment. In view of his young age, they wished to avoid midfoot fusion and proceeded to surgery via a direct dorsal approach.

The cartilage was excised between the adjoining surfaces. Fixation was obtained with a 3.5 mm cannulated screw, supplemented with synthetic calcium phosphate graft. Complete bony union ensued at 3 months postoperatively with complete resolution of pain. He remained pain-free at 1 year's follow-up having returned to normal activities. Bony union was not confirmed by CT scan.

Some believe bipartite navicular, a relatively uncommon occurrence encountered in young children, constitutes an aetiological factor in the development of Müller-Weiss disease. On the other hand, Yamaguchi et al. believe that a bipartite navicular results from failure of fusion of two or more ossification centers and is a completely different entity from Müller-Weiss disease. Since the latter had been described mainly in middle-aged adults, they argued that the 14-year-old boy in Doyle et al.'s series (2012) represented a case of bipartite navicular and not of Müller-Weiss disease, while cognizant of the fact there were no details given of the boy other than that he was treated conservatively (Doyle et al. 2012). In fact, the adolescent boy had presented with a 'fracture' at the lateral corner of a laterally compressed navicular following a football injury. Unaware of the condition of Müller-Weiss disease at that time, the author had considered open reduction and internal fixation. The lateral fragment was very small and the author would most probably have encountered the same disappointing problem of nonunion as Yamaguchi et al. Fortunately, his symptoms settled within 3 months and he has remained asymptomatic since until the age of 29 years old. He now faces talonaviculocuneiform arthrodesis surgery.

Both of Yamaguchi et al.'s cases are classic examples of Müller-Weiss disease with a comma-shaped navicular, compression and fragmentation of the lateral part, and dorsal extrusion of the lateral fragment. Although there is some degree of medial extrusion of the navicular pole, medial talonavicular subluxation does not appear marked. Their first illustration suggests there is abduction at the midfoot. However, this cannot be ascertained as only the midfoot region is shown and not the entire foot. If correct, this adolescent pattern would match that shown by Ahmed et al. (2019).

Both feet of Yamaguchi et al. had early-onset Group 1 Müller-Weiss disease that were operated upon for presumed bipartite naviculars.

## 12.2 Osteochondritis of the Navicular

Sharp et al. (Brisbane, Australia, (2003) reported on a 17-year-old boy with presumed bilateral osteochondritis of the navicular (Sharp et al. 2003). Initial radiographs at the age of 12 years were construed as having shown features consistent with Köhler's disease. He was treated nonoperatively. Repeat radiographs obtained 5 years later were then deemed to have demonstrated features consistent with Brailsford's disease.

The authors pointed out that there were no documented cases of Köhler's disease with clinical and radiological abnormalities persisting into adulthood. Nor were there, at the time of writing, cases of Brailsford's disease having had abnormalities in childhood. They hypothesized that perhaps a late onset of Köhler's disease in their patient might not have allowed enough time for remodeling to take place, resulting in misshapen and extruded naviculars. They did not deem it 'realistic' either that the feet could have changed from Köhler's disease at the age of 12 years to Brailsford's disease at skeletal maturity. Their case fitted neither into the category of Köhler's disease, which affects a much younger age and resolves spontaneously. Nor did it fit into that of Brailsford's disease, which affects the lateral navicular at a much older age. They concluded that, since their patient fitted into neither category, they must have encountered a new condition occurring in teenage years. They opined that their patient represented a case of osteochondritis of the navicular bone with symptoms persisting into skeletal maturity.

The radiographs at the age of 12 years already demonstrated the characteristic changes of Müller-Weiss disease with a comma-shaped navicular, compression and fragmentation of the lateral portions and dorsal extrusion of the lateral navicular fragments. Of the radiographs obtained at the age of 17 years, only the lateral standing views of the feet and ankles were shown. They were no different from those at the age of 12 years.

Both feet of Sharp et al. had early-onset Group 1 Müller-Weiss disease that were treated for presumed osteochondritis of the navicular.

## 12.3 Crank-Shaped Arthrodesis for Flatfoot with Bipartite Navicular

Tanaka et al. (Japan, (2006) published a case report describing creation of a crank-shaped talo-cuneiform articulation to preserve midfoot motion in a 44-year-old recreational tennis player with bipartite navicular, flatfoot deformity and talonavicular arthritis (Tanaka et al. 2006). They used the terms bipartite navicular, aseptic necrosis of the navicular, osteochondrosis of the navicular and Müller-Weiss disease synonymously. The patient had been aware of a bony protrusion over the dorsum of the left foot since the age of 21 years, but only became symptomatic two weeks prior to attendance.

Dorsoplantar weight-bearing radiograph was interpreted as having shown lateral displacement of a dorsal fragment, which appeared superimposed over the second and third cuneiforms. The medial navicular fragment was subluxed medially and inferiorly. On lateral standing radiograph, the medial arch sagged and the lateral fragment was displaced dorsally. Lateral tomography revealed a cyst in the talar head and neck with marked degeneration at the talonavicular joint.

Analysis of the provided radiographs reveals advanced talonavicular arthritis, a comma-shaped navicular with marked compression and fragmentation of its lateral portion, dorsolateral displacement of the lateral navicular fragment with direct articulation of the talar head with the lateral cuneiform bone. Apparent medial extrusion of the medial navicular pole is due to midfoot abduction, as there is no real medial talonavicular subluxation. The forefoot is not well visualized, but the second ray appears to be longer. In some but not all ways, these features resemble the pattern encountered by Ahmed et al. in Egyptian adolescents but at a later more advanced stage with arthritis more marked at the talonavicular joint (Ahmed et al. 2019).

After failure to improve with an arch support for 2 months, surgery was embarked upon. The talonavicular joint was exposed and prepared via a medial incision. The articular cartilage at the lateral portion of the talar head was preserved. The dorsally extruded lateral navicular fragment was approached through a dorsolateral incision. One centimeter was excised off it to create a new pseudo joint between it and the lateral talar head with no interpositional material.

The medial navicular fragment was arthrodesed to the talar head with 3 partially threaded AO screws. The lateral navicular fragment was fused to the lateral cuneiform with 2 partially threaded AO screws. All hardware was subsequently removed at 2 years following surgery. At 5 years' final follow-up, the patient was able to play tennis twice a week without pain. Dorsiflexion and plantarflexion were equal on either side. Inversion was 25° on the operated side compared to 50° on the unoperated side. Lateral radiographs obtained in maximum plantarflexion demonstrated preservation of 6° of motion at the crank-shaped joint compared to 9° at the opposite talonavicular articulation. Méary's angle improved from 12° to 7° while calcaneal pitch increased from 12° to 14°.

The authors concluded that their novel crank-shaped joint between the lateral part of the talar head and fused lateral navicular fragment-to-lateral cuneiform bone mass preserved movement compared to motion-sacrificing talonavicular, triple or talonaviculocuneiform arthrodesis.

Their case represented a Wong Group 3B Maceira Stage V with dorsal extrusion of the lateral navicular fragment and formation of a talocuneiform articulation. In all probability, the patient's pain was relieved by the arthrodesis performed between the talar head and medial navicular remnant. The authors believed that fusing the dorsally displaced lateral navicular fragment to the nearby lateral cuneiform bone with which the talar head was already articulating, preserved some degree of midfoot motion.

## 12.4 Talonavicular Arthrodesis and Excision of the Dorsally Extruded Lateral Fragment

Chujo et al. (Hiroshima, Japan, (2023) reported on a 13-year-old boy with flatfoot, midfoot abduction and a so-called bipartite navicular (Chujo et al. 2023). CT scan demonstrated dorsal extrusion of the lateral navicular fragment and medial and plantar displacement of the medial navicular fragment.

Following failed nonoperative treatment, he proceeded to surgery via a dorsal incision. The dorsally extruded lateral navicular fragment was excised. The severely arthritic remaining medial talonavicular joint was prepared. The medial navicular fragment was lifted upwards and pushed laterally to restore the medial arch. Talonavicular arthrodesis was stabilized with a cannulated 4.0 mm cancellous screw and a compression staple. Cancellous bone, harvested from the medial malleolus, filled the lateral defect resulting from excision of the lateral navicular fragment.

Dorsoplantar talo-first metatarsal angle improved from −35° to −7°. Méary's angle improved from −28° to −8°. Calcaneal pitch increased from 8° to 12°. The talonavicular arthrodesis united with complete resolution of pain. The patient returned to playing basketball six months after surgery.

Postoperative radiographs demonstrate presence of a joint space at the level of the lateral naviculocuneiform articulation, although the joint surfaces appear slightly irregular especially at the navicular side. The surface of the lateral talar head as well as the lateral surface of the medial navicular remnant have been prepared as evidenced by the presence of fenestration drill holes on the intraoperative photographs. Cancellous bone graft, inserted in the lateral defect between these prepared surfaces, was stopped short of the unprepared proximal surfaces of the lateral cuneiform and part of the middle cuneiform distally by a retractor. The talonavicular arthrodesis united as did the graft to the talar head and medial navicular fragments. A pseudo articulation must have formed at the lateral naviculocuneiform joint space.

**Concluding Remarks**

This Chapter drives home lessons to be learnt from past cases of Müller-Weiss disease treated for presumed bipartite navicular.

Poor outcomes reported by Yamaguchi et al. (2016) following open reduction and internal fixation of the so-called bipartite navicular reinforce Fernández de Retana et al.'s previous warning regarding the lateral navicular fragment in Müller-Weiss disease being too small for fixation and not having enough viable bone for bone healing to proceed (Fernández de Retana et al. 2004).

Both Tanaka et al. and Chujo et al. performed talonavicular arthrodesis (Tanaka et al. 2006; Chujo et al. 2023). While Chujo et al. excised the displaced dorsolateral navicular fragment, (2023) Tanaka et al. instead fused it to the lateral cuneiform (Tanaka et al. 2006). The resulting crank-shaped joint between the lateral part of the talar head and fused lateral navicular fragment–to-lateral cuneiform bone mass purportedly served to preserve midfoot motion.

In all likelihood, the talonavicular arthrodesis component probably contributed the most to relieving pain in both cases. Equally good outcomes followed either excision of the lateral navicular fragment or its fusion to the lateral cuneiform bone.

## References

Ahmed AA, Kandil MI, Tabl EA. Preliminary outcomes of calcaneal lengthening in adolescent flatfoot in Müller-Weiss disease. Foot Ankle Int. 2019;40(7):803–807. https://doi.org/10.1177/1071100719833928

Alomran D, Gaber K, Kishta W. Mueller-Weiss syndrome, An unexpected cause of mid foot pain in adolescents. J Orthop Reports. 2024;3(1):1–5. https://doi.org/10.1016/j.jorep.2023.100240.

Chujo T, Nakasa T, Ikuta Y, Kawabata S, Adachi N. Talonavicular arthrodesis using a screw and compression staple in a patient with bipartite navicular bone: a case report. Cureus. 2023;15(8): e43122. https://doi.org/10.7759/cureus.43122.

Doyle T, Napier RJ, Wong-Chung J. Recognition and management of Müller-Weiss disease. Foot Ankle Int. 2012;33(4):275–81. https://doi.org/10.3113/FAI.2012.0275.

Fernández de Retana P, Maceira E, Fernández-Valencia JA, Suso S. Arthrodesis of the talonavicular-cuneiform joints in Müller-Weiss disease. Foot Ankle Clin. 2004;9(1):65–72. https://doi.org/10.1016/S1083-7515(03)00175-X

Sharp RJ, Calder JD, Saxby TS. Osteochondritis of the navicular: a case report. Foot Ankle Int. 2003;24(6):509–13. https://doi.org/10.1177/107110070302400611.

Tanaka Y, Takakura Y, Omokawa S, Kumai T, Sugimoto K. Crank-shaped arthrodesis for a flatfoot with a bipartite navicular: a case report. Foot Ankle Int. 2006;27(9):734–7. https://doi.org/10.1177/107110070602700914.

Yamaguchi S, Niki H, Akagi R, Yamamoto Y, Sasho T. Failure of internal fixation for painful bipartite navicular in two adolescent soccer players: a report of two cases. J Foot Ankle Surg. 2016;55(6):1323–6. https://doi.org/10.1053/j.jfas.2016.01.015.

# Part III
# The Future of Looking Back

# Chapter 13
# Müller-Weiss Disease: Past, Present and Future Directions

**Abstract** A century later, much remains to be discovered about Müller-Weiss disease. Although an index minus metatarsal formula plays an important role, other aetiological factors are yet to be identified. It is not known when disease actually begins for lack of earlier radiographs that predate disease detection. Geographical variations such as early-onset disease in Egypt, different Müller-Weissoid and reverse Müller-Weissoid patterns in Spain and Northern Ireland, exist which require elucidation. The catchy term paradoxical pes planus varus only applies when both flatfoot and heel varus are present. WBCT may reveal why heels do not always varize while the talar head displaces laterally. Results of pedobarography should be reported according to the Wong Groups. Future research should look into possibility of preserving some or all of the naviculocuneiform joints, the role of shortening metatarsal osteotomies and how to proceed once fracture occurs at the lateral navicular, be it undisplaced or displaced. Proposed novel surgical procedures such as navicular replacement require close scrutiny. A combination of the Wong Groups and Maceira stages may provide a common platform for disease reporting and measuring outcomes of nonoperative treatment and various surgical procedures in controlled fashion. Only then can gold standards of treatment be clearly defined.

**Keywords** Müller-Weiss disease · Epidemiology · Aetiology · Classifications · Metatarsal shortening osteotomy · Navicular replacement

## Introduction

This last chapter highlights the challenges and controversies surrounding the knowns and unknowns of this condition. Although it raises many more questions than it does give answers, hopefully it will provide the stimulus to discovering the correct answers and help lift Müller-Weiss disease out of obscurity.

> …there are known knowns; there are things we know we know. We also know there are known unknowns; that is to say we know there are some things we do not know. But there are also unknown unknowns — the ones we don't know we don't know.
>
> Donald Rumsfeld, 2002

© The Author(s), under exclusive license to Springer Nature Switzerland AG 2024 
J. Wong-Chung, *Comprehensive Guide to Müller-Weiss Disease*,
https://doi.org/10.1007/978-3-031-66644-5_13

## 13.1 Geographical Distribution

Whilst the early literature on Müller-Weiss disease emerged from Europe with an apparent preponderance in Spain (Maceira and Rochera 2004), clusters are being increasingly reported throughout the world. For instance, the recent study of 95 feet from Northern Ireland (Wong-Chung et al. 2023) represents one of the world's largest series outside of Spain. It is tempting to speculate that the landfall of the Spanish Armada off the west coast of Ireland may have contributed to this high incidence. One Northern Irish patient with bilateral disease volunteered to obtain DNA testing from Ancestry.com. It revealed that she was 95% Irish with no Spanish connection. Furthermore, large surgical series continue to emanate from China (Zhang and Yu 2018; Yuan et al. 2019) and Thailand (Harnroongroj et al. 2021). Any further plans to trace ancestry in the other 93 feet were therefore abandoned.

For reasons unknown, literature on the subject remains scarce from South (Molina et al. 2023) and North America. At the time of writing, Foot and Ankle International journal contained only 9 articles on Müller-Weiss disease, none of which emanated from the USA. Two originated from China (Yuan et al. 2019; Cao et al. 2012), and 1 each from Japan (Tanaka et al. 2006), Thailand (Harnroongroj et al. 2021), Israel (Hetsroni et al. 2007), Egypt (Ahmed et al. 2019a; Ahmed et al. b), Switzerland (Fornaciari et al. 2014), Spain (Li et al. 2017) and Northern Ireland (Doyle et al. 2012). The Journal of Foot and Ankle Surgery also held 9 articles, 1 each from Japan (Yamaguchi et al. 2016), Taiwan (Chang et al. 2019), China (Yu et al. 2012), Thailand (Harnroongroj and Chuckpaiwong 2018), Turkey (Tosun et al. 2011), Egypt (Chiavegatti et al. 2018), Holland (Tan et al. 2011) and 2 case reports from Colorado and California, USA (Toren et al. 2013; Nelson and Rivello 2012).

The oldest specimen, 2300 years old, has been unearthed in Egypt (Chiavegatti et al. 2018). Contemporary Egyptian surgeons report a reverse type of Müller-Weiss disease, in which the disease affects the naviculocuneiform more than the talonavicular joint in adolescents (Ahmed et al. 2019b). Contrary to the recommendations of Li, Myerson, Monteagudo and Maceira (Li et al. 2017), the Egyptian adolescent feet had a lateral column lengthening instead of a lateral displacement calcaneal osteotomy (See also Chap. 4 Sect. 4.6.1).

Monteagudo and Maceira had defined Müller-Weissoid changes as disease developing in late adulthood in naviculars that had previously been normal radiologically in "young adults" (Monteagudo and Maceira 2019). However, they did not specify which joints were most affected. Out of 95 feet, Wong-Chung et al. identified 26 (27.4%) naviculars that developed disease having been normal radiologically 6.8 years earlier (Wong-Chung et al. 2023). In 23 of the 26 (88.5%), compression and arthritis affected the talonavicular joint predominantly and were termed Müller-Weissoid feet. The naviculocuneiform joint was more affected in the other 3 (11.5%), which were designated as "reverse Müller-Weissoid" feet. The example shown by Monteagudo and Maceira fits with the reverse Müller-Weissoid category with identical radiographic features to those of Wong-Chung et al. (See also Chap. 4 on Classification Sect. 4.7). Unfortunately, Monteagudo and Maceira did not disclose the number of feet with reverse Müller-Weissoid disease, nor is it known whether they had encountered any Müller-Weissoid disease as defined by Wong-Chung et al. Geographical differences in pattern of the disease may thus exist, which require further analysis.

## 13.2 Age and Gender

Consensus exists on predominance of the condition in females, although the actual female to male ratio varies widely. While it tends to manifest mostly during the fifth and sixth decades of life, there are increasing reports of early-onset disease (Wong-Chung et al. 2023; Ahmed et al. 2019b).

## 13.3 Aetiology

Many theories have been put forward regarding aetiology of the disease since it was first described in 1927 by Müller (1927) and Weiss (1927). Much of what is known comes from the extensive studies by Maceira (Maceira and Rochera 2004) and Monteagudo (Monteagudo and Maceira 2019). These investigators initially thought that delayed ossification of the navicular, brought about by famine from the Spanish civil war, played as important a role as lateral shift in distribution of compression forces arising from a short first ray. However, other authors do not share the same experience of a past history of environmental or nutritional stress in their patients (Doyle et al. 2012). More recently, even Monteagudo and Maceira also remarked that, apart from an occasional new attendance from the era of the famine, their recent new patients have not suffered any such previous stress (Monteagudo and Maceira 2019).

Overall, there is scholarly agreement upon a mechanical factor in the development of the disease, namely brachymetatarsia of the first ray which leads to a shift of compression forces to the lateral part of the navicular. A long second ray appears to be a common denominator amongst all the groups and subgroups of Wong-Chung et al. (2023). The longer second metatarsal was noticed even as far back as 1939 by Brailsford (1939).

At this stage, it would be appropriate to acknowledge the important contributions of our predecessors Brailsford, who likened the condition to osteochondritis of the medial femoral condyle and Volk (1937), who introduced the term bipartite navicular (See also Chap. 1 on Aetiology to Nomenclature) (Brailsford 1939; Volk 1937).

*Known Known & Known Unknowns*: It is known that feet with Müller-Weiss disease tend to have an index minus metatarsal formula. But many more feet with such a Morton's type morphology do not develop Müller-Weiss disease. And of those who do, why do some manifest at an early age and others at a much later age in their fifth to sixth decades? To compound issues, except for the Müller-Weissoid feet, it is not known when the disease actually starts because earliest radiographs demonstrating normality are not available.

In summary, while a longer second metatarsal is accepted as an important factor in the pathogenesis of the condition, it is not known what triggers development of Müller-Weiss disease in some naviculars while others continue as normal. Nutritional deficiency, as originally hypothesized by Maceira and Rochera to be a major factor, no longer seems to be a responsible ingredient in contemporary times. Excessive stress on the foot at an early age as in child athletes may play a role but does not explain the incidence in many more other affected non-athletes.

## 13.4 Parallels with Navicular Stress Fractures

Navicular stress fractures were first described in 1958 in the outer front and rear limbs of racing dogs (Bateman 1958). The right hindfoot is most often involved, because the dogs run counterclockwise on banked tracks and exert greater muscular forces on the bones of the uphill foot to maintain traction while constantly turning left. It was not until 12 years later that human case reports were first published in 2 high school boys by Towne et al. (1970).

The injury often passes underdiagnosed and requires special imaging for diagnosis (Goergen et al. 1981; Hunter 1981; Pavlov et al. 1983). Mohiuddin et al. even believe there is a strong possibility that Müller-Weiss disease is a sequel of undiagnosed navicular stress fractures (Mohiuddin et al. 2014).

Certain differences in pattern and location of fracture between Müller-Weiss disease and stress injuries are worth mentioning. Whereas the sagittal cleft runs from dorsal distal to plantar proximal in Müller-Weiss disease (Maceira and Rochera 2004), stress fractures begin at the proximal dorsal articular surface and propagates distally and plantar in the sagittal plane, in a slightly oblique medial to lateral direction, as the injury progresses (Saxena et al. 2000). In Müller-Weiss disease, fragmentation takes place more commonly at the level of the lateral cuneiform bone or lateral intercuneiform joint (Wong-Chung et al. 2021). On the other hand, stress fracture is classically described in the central third of the bone at the level of the intermediate cuneiform bone, just lateral to the center of the talar head (Torg et al. 1982; Mann and Pedowitz 2009). Bilaterality is rare in stress fractures but common in Müller-Weiss disease. The latter tends to affect women in their fifth to sixth decades of life, whereas stress fractures are associated with explosive athletic activities such as sprinting, jumping and hurdling, nearly always affecting the take-off leg (Fitch et al. 1989).

In the differential diagnosis of navicular stress fractures, Monteagudo and Martínez-de-Albornoz nicknamed Müller-Weiss disease the "mimic navicular fracture" (Monteagudo and Martínez-de-Albornoz 2022). They recommended ruling out the latter clinically by the presence of a paradoxical flatfoot and radiologically by evidence of navicular dysplasia.

Torg et al. have attributed predilection of the central third of the navicular for stress fractures to its relative avascularity. Using a Spälteholz technique in only 5 adult cadavers, they demonstrated that multiple blood vessels entered the navicular from the nonarticular medial and lateral cortices and extended centripetally into the bone, leaving the central one-third relatively devoid of vascular supply (Torg et al. 1982).

However, using a modified Spälteholz techniquet, McKeon et al. found a dense intraosseous vascular supply throughout the navicular with no avascular regions in 30 of 51 (58.8%) cadaveric feet (McKeon et al. 2012). While an avascular zone was identified in 21 (41.2%) specimens, only 6 (11.8%) had an avascular central zone extending to the central dorsal cortex, the region where most navicular stress fractures originate. In 2 feet (3.9%), a central avascular zone extended to the dorsolateral surface. In 10 feet, an avascular zone present in the central region did not extend to the dorsal surface (19.6%) and 3 specimens (5.9%) had an avascular zone in the plantar region of the bone only.

The authors concluded that a consistent central zone of avascularity was not identified in the majority of their specimens with only 11.8% of cadavers having a central avascular region that extended to the dorsal surface of the bone, where stress fractures usually begin. Others had zones of relative avascularity in regions that are not typically associated with stress fractures. While an area of relative avascularity in the dorsal central third of the navicular may contribute to stress fracture in some athletes, it is not known whether all athletes have avascular regions within their navicular bone.

Fitch et al. had noted that a large number of patients with stress fractures had a short first metatarsal and relatively longer second metatarsal. This anatomical variation would subject the lateral portion of the navicular to higher shear stresses. Metatarsal adduction and pronation would further increase forces acting upon the lateral navicular during weight-bearing and lift-off, rendering it more susceptible to injury (Fitch et al. 1989). Pavlov et al. had also noticed this index minus configuration as well as metatarsus adductus in association with stress fractures (Pavlov et al. 1983). Of all the risk factors proposed for stress fractures such as calcaneal pitch angle, Méary's angle, pes cavus, pronation velocity, medial narrowing of the talonavicular joint space, talar beaking, limited ankle dorsiflexion, short first metatarsal and metatarsus adductus, none have reached statistical significance (Coris and Lombardo 2003).

### *13.4.1 Prophylactic or Therapeutic Shortening Metatarsal Osteomies for Navicular Stress Fractures and Müller-Weiss Disease*

Interestingly, for both navicular stress fractures and Müller-Weiss disease, scholars have reached the same conclusion of a biomechanical imbalance created by a short first or longer second metatarsal generating abnormal shear stress at the lateral portion of the navicular. Yet, there is no mention in the literature of shortening metatarsal osteotomies either as primary or as prophylactic treatment for stress fractures or Müller-Weiss disease. To alleviate pain symptoms in Müller-Weiss disease, Li et al. have performed lateral displacement calcaneal osteotomy to shift forces from lateral to medial (Li et al. 2017). However, even though investigators are aware of the index minus configuration in their patients, no one has considered the idea of performing shortening metatarsal osteotomies to decrease forces acting upon the lateral navicular in Müller-Weiss disease. Nor in the case of stress fractures has shortening metatarsal surgery been considered either as part of surgical treatment to promote union, in the treatment of delayed and nonunion which are commonly encountered, in the prevention of recurrence of stress fracture or to address persistent pain despite radiological union following nonoperative or surgical fixation. This line of approach may warrant further investigation.

Despite any shared features, it is important not to mistake Müller-Weiss disease for a navicular stress fracture. Each has its own characteristics as outlined above. Each behaves differently and treatment strategies differ.

### *13.4.2 Stress Fracture of Second Metatarsal Following Talonavicular Arthrodesis*

Cullen et al. reported a case of stress fracture of the second metatarsal diaphysis at 18 months following successful talonavicular arthrodesis for Müller-Weiss disease in a 34-year-old male accountant (Cullen et al. 2005). There was no history of injury. He walked 30 minutes to and from work every day. After 7 months of failed nonoperative measures, he underwent bone grafting and plating, which led to bony union.

No preoperative radiographs were made available for review. The second metatarsal actually looked shorter than the first on dorsoplantar radiograph. The authors hypothesized that altered mechanics following talonavicular arthrodesis somehow led to increased load across the second ray.

## 13.5 The Term "Paradoxical Pes Planus Varus"

Has the time arrived to restrict use of this appellation? Coined by Maceira and Rochera in 2004, the term "paradoxical pes planus varus" has perpetuated the notion that the heel is always in varus in Müller-Weiss disease (Maceira and Rochera 2004). So much so, that some authorities declare that if the heel is not in varus, it is not Müller-Weiss disease!

This topic has been expounded upon at length in the previous Chapters on Clinical Features, Radiographic Features and Classification Systems. To summarize, the points for and against universal use of the term are:

- According to Maceira's own classification, the arch is raised in Stage II, and neutral in Stages I and III. The medial arch sags in Stages IV and V only.
- In an extensive radiographic analysis of 68 feet, Wong-Chung et al. found the heel to be in varus in only 33% (Wong-Chung et al. 2021).
- The combination of heel varus and medial arch sag, which would fit the description of 'paradoxical pes planus varus', was present in just 26%.
- The commonest combination was of heel valgus and medial arch sag in 56%.
- Several other investigators have also reported that the heel is not always in varus.
- Indeed, Ahmed et al. performed lateral column lengthening in 13 adolescent feet with Müller-Weiss disease (Ahmed et al. 2019b).
- How did this notion of universal heel varus happen? Looking at the illustrations of Maceira and Rochera (2004) in 2004 and again at those of Monteagudo and Maceira (2019) in 2019, heel varus was judged by looking at the heels from above knee level. In fact, the photographs taken at ankle level reveal negative peekaboo signs and the still shots from the back show heel valgus. Viewed from an elevated height, all heels will give a false positive peekaboo sign (Manoli et al. 1993; Manoli and Graham 2005).
- Furthermore, in their original description, Maceira and Monteagudo acknowledged that subtle heel varus can be difficult to detect and recommended palpation of the heel during heel rise (Monteagudo and Maceira 2019). Again, most heels will go into varus when standing on tiptoes. A better clinical way of assessing heel varus is to hold the heel in the palm of the hand with the patient sitting or supine and the ankle held in dorsiflexion.
- Also, based on the concept of the 'coxa pedis', Maceira and Rochera inferred that the heel must move into varus as the talar head shifts laterally. While the corollary applies, namely that the heel usually moves into valgus when the talar head shifts medially as in classic progressive collapsing foot deformity (PCFD), Maceira's assumption may not be necessarily correct and warrants further investigation with weight-bearing CT (WBCT).
- Like in a chain reaction, a recent literature review, quoting Monteagudo and Maceira, also recommended assessing heel varus during heel rise and endorsed the concept of obligatory heel varus because the talar head moves laterally (Hermena and Francis 2021).
- Surgeons who perform lateral displacement calcaneal osteotomy alone (Li et al. 2017) in the treatment of Müller-Weiss disease should confirm that the heel is actually in varus by correctly obtained Saltzman's radiographic hindfoot alignment views (Saltzman and el-Khoury 1995).

Conclusion: Based on the foregoing points, use of the term 'paradoxical pes planus varus' needs to be restricted to when all of its described components are present. Perhaps even, the time may have come to stop using the term altogether, because it only perpetuates the incorrect belief among radiologists and physicians that the heel must always be in varus in Müller-Weiss disease regardless of its stage.

## 13.6 Classification Systems in Müller-Weiss Disease

- Maceira and Rochera's five-stage classification is based on Méary's angle alone (2004) (Maceira and Rochera 2004).
- Even Monteagudo and Maceira (2019) acknowledge that, while it may be useful for descriptive purposes to explain pathomechanics of the condition, neither does it serve as guide to treatment nor does it have prognostic value.
- Mayich's modification (2016) to characterize Maceira Stage IV by the presence of subtalar arthritis has not gained support (Mayich 2016).
- Stage V of Maceira's classification remains a useful landmark because it marks end-stage disease with a definite end-point, denoted by direct articulation of the talar head with the lateral cuneiform bone.
- Monteagudo and Maceira (2019) elaborated on two terms, the second of which had barely received mention in 2004, and introduced yet another appellation. The first *epidemic* group describes disease presumed to have been caused by the famine of the Spanish civil war. In these so-called 'children of war', nutritional deficiency led to delay in ossification, which in turn predisposed the weakened navicular to deform under eccentric stress from an overlong second metatarsal. The second *non-epidemic* group has no known history of nutritional or environmental stress. Disease is said to develop in child athletes with short first metatarsals and healthy naviculars subjected to 'too much stress, too soon'. Although the authors maintain that Müller-Weiss disease begins in childhood, they introduce a third group called *Müller-Weissoid* to describe Müller-Weiss changes occurring in late adulthood in naviculars which were known to be radiologically normal in early adulthood.
- Harnroongroj and Chuckpaiwong (2021) recommended that future classifications should take into account two descriptive factors, namely the presence of talonavicular arthritis and the dorsoplantar talo-first metatarsal (DPTFM) angle (Harnroongroj et al. 2021). According to their experience, talonavicular arthritis and midfoot abduction with a DPTFM angle of greater than 13° indicate likelihood of failure of nonoperative treatment and the need for surgery.
- The parameters taken into account by Wong-Chung et al. (2023) when formulating their groups included both descriptive factors: (a) age of onset (b) joints affected (c) previous radiologically normal navicular (d) lateral Méary's angle and (e) dorsoplantar talo-first metatarsal angle. With any of the groups or subgroups, the subtalar ± calcaneocuboid joint may or may not be involved. In considering the joints affected, the authors instead distinguish between affection of the talonavicular joint only and involvement of both talonavicular and naviculocuneiform joints, notably in their Group 3. Group 1 early-onset disease occurred in the youngest 9 to 29-year-old patients, none of whom has required surgery yet. It had the greatest degree of medial extrusion, highest degree of compression at

the lateral naviculocuneiform (NC) joint and the lowest Kite's angles. All were index negative and had a fracture at the lateral corner of the navicular except for one. Group 2 late-onset Müller-Weissoid disease occurred in patients in their sixth decade having had a radiologically normal navicular, on average 6.7 years earlier. These feet had the lowest degree of medial extrusion, the lowest degree of compression at NC2 and NC3, the highest Kite's angles and lowest degree of overlength of the second metatarsal. None had complete fracture except for 1 infraction seen on CT scan but not visualized at surgery. Degeneration took place mostly at the talonavicular joint with early changes at NC3 in 48%. Surgical treatment consisted of talonavicular ± subtalar arthrodesis. Group 3 late-onset disease in adults with no previous documentation of a radiologically normal navicular was subdivided into 3 subgroups. Group 3A affects the talonavicular joint only with no involvement of the naviculocuneiform joint. It had no fracture except for one infraction. Surgery consisted of talonavicular ± subtalar arthrodesis. Disease in Group 3B and 3C affects both sides of the navicular. Group 3B, in which the talonavicular is more affected than the naviculocuneiform joints, had the greatest incidence of Maceira Stage V disease. Group 3C, in which the naviculocuneiform is more affected than the talonaviculocuneiform joint, is termed 'reverse Müller-Weiss disease'. It had the greatest degree of midfoot abduction and overlength of the second metatarsal. Fracture of the lateral navicular occurred in 65% of Group 3B and 32% of Group 3C. Surgery in both Groups 3B and 3C consisted of talonaviculocuneiform arthrodesis plus an interpositional tricortical iliac crest bone graft in case of fracture or inadequate bone stock at the lateral navicular (See also Chap. 4 on Classification Systems).

- A combination of Maceira's staging and Wong-Chung's grouping may prove a more beneficial and useful platform for reporting results of nonoperative and operative treatment:
- For instance, common straightforward presentations are (1) Group 2 Müller-Weissoid disease involving mostly the talonavicular joint and (2) Group 3A late-onset involving the talonavicular joint only. Any of the aforesaid groups may be at various Maceira Stages II, III or IV. Stage V was not encountered in either of these 2 groups.
- A frequently shown illustration of a more complicated case in the literature is of a Wong Group 3B Maceira Stage V, where the talonavicular joint is more affected than the naviculocuneiform joint, with fracture and dorsal extrusion of the lateral navicular fragment, pronounced medial talonavicular subluxation and direct articulation of the talar head with the lateral cuneiform—the talocuneiform articulation.
- Less common presentations in the literature but of no lesser importance are the Group 3C 'reverse Müller-Weiss' cases, which deserve further in-depth multicenter investigation.
- And then there are also the Group 3B feet at various Maceira Stages II, III or IV.

Most studies in the literature just put cases from all groups together when reporting results of surgical treatment, thereby creating confounding variables akin to comparing apples and oranges mixed together (Tile 1988, 1995).

### *13.6.1 Müller-Weiss Disease with Concomitant Asymmetric Varus Ankle Osteoarthritis*

Of the 37 feet that underwent surgery in the case series of Wong-Chung et al. (2021), 3 had associated asymmetric varus ankle osteoarthritis. One patient underwent bilateral pantalar arthrodesis 7 years apart. In the other, the talonavicular joint was not painful and total ankle arthroplasty was combined with lateral displacement calcaneal osteotomy to correct heel varus.

Asymmetric varus ankle osteoarthritis may represent a further stage of the disease caused by prolonged heel varus in certain cases.

Interestingly, a recent review article by Angthong et al. (2023) included the aforementioned 2021 article of Wong-Chung et al. The authors drew up a treatment algorithm. The last limb of their decision flowchart includes options of total ankle arthroplasty or ankle arthrodesis combined with subtalar and talonavicular, triple or talonaviculocuneiform fusion for late-stage disease involving the ankle.

## 13.7 Significance of the Dorsoplantar Talo-First Metatarsal Angle in Müller-Weiss Disease

Harnroongroj and Chuckpaiwong had recommended that any future classification should take into account the dorsoplantar talo-first metatarsal angle (Harnroongroj et al. 2021). Group 3C reverse Müller-Weiss disease had the highest degree of midfoot abduction, as measured by the dorsoplantar talo-first metatarsal angle, and also the greatest overlength of the second metatarsal (Wong-Chung et al. 2023).

A strong correlation existed between the lateral Méary's angle and the dorsoplantar talo-first metatarsal angle ($P < 0.001$). However, unlike Harnroongroj and Chuckpaiwong who had found that midfoot abduction of greater than 13° indicated the need for operative intervention, Wong-Chung et al. did not share the same experience in 37 of 95 feet that failed nonoperative treatment and proceeded to surgery (Wong-Chung et al. 2023). The DPTFM angles averaged -4° in the operated group and -5° in the nonoperated group, negative value denoting midfoot abduction ($p = 0.928$).

## 13.8 Surgery in Müller-Weiss Disease

Harnroongroj and Chuckpaiwong remarked upon the good results reported following all kinds of surgery ranging from percutaneous decompression to bone grafting in early-stage disease without collapse of the navicular bone, and from talonavicular and triple arthrodesis to perinavicular arthrodesis in later stages (Harnroongroj and Chuckpaiwong 2018). "All these techniques have demonstrated satisfactory outcomes. However, the study limitations have included small sample sizes, short follow-up periods, and a lack of in-depth radiographic details."

The previous statement is reminiscent of an era when many operations in flatfoot surgery seemed to all work well.

> "Nothing elicits controversy as much as the 'appropriate' correction of flatfoot. To some extent, this controversy has to do with the many satisfactory operations that are available for correction of similar deformity." (Myerson 2005)

On the surface, different procedures appear to work equally well in Müller-Weiss disease. But determining the optimum procedure for the individual case is a different matter. Let us first summarize the currently performed operations and then consider some of the many unknown factors in surgery for Müller-Weiss disease.

### *13.8.1 Overview of Current Surgery in Müller-Weiss Disease*

- **Talonaviculocuneiform Arthrodesis for All**: Fernández de Retana, Maceira et al. (2004) acknowledged the lack of a surgical gold standard and argued the case for universal talonaviculocuneiform arthrodesis (Fernández de Retana et al. 2004). Open reduction and internal fixation were not feasible, as the lateral navicular fragment was often too small. They advised against talonavicular and triple arthrodesis as they did not address disease at the naviculocuneiform joints. Of note, they only included the medial naviculocuneiform (NC1) joint in the fusion mass, *leaving NC2 and NC3 unprepared*. Cao HH et al. have followed suit, adding a reverse V-shaped plantar closing wedge through the talonavicular joint to correct the medial arch. They also *left NC2 and NC3 untouched* (Cao et al. 2012, 2017).
- **Talonavicular Arthrodesis with Reduction of Medial Talonavicular Subluxation**: Fornaciari et al. recommended reduction using a lateral tension band principle (Fornaciari et al. 2014). Yuan et al. claimed ability to perform talonavicular arthrodesis even in the most severe cases of medial talonavicular subluxation, by utilizing a pin distractor to laterally derotate the navicular from its medially subluxed position (Yuan et al. 2019). They resorted to talonaviculocuneiform arthrodesis only in the presence of associated severe naviculocuneiform arthritis, in which case they arthrodesed the talonavicular and medial naviculocuneiform (NC1) joint only, *leaving NC2 and NC3 untouched.*
- **Talonaviculocuneiform Arthrodesis with Reduction of Medial Talonavicular Subluxation**: Bai et al. believe that shortening and sagging of the medial column

are all due to medial subluxation of the navicular (Bai et al. 2023). They therefore advocate that the navicular should be repositioned from its plantar and medial subluxated position to its correct location at the apex of the medial longitudinal arch, thereby simultaneously correcting both medial column length and medial arch sag. In addition to an extensive medial release, excision of any lateral blockages as also advised by Nelson and Rivello is necessary to obtain reduction (Nelson and Rivello 2012). Any lateral defect can then be filled with tricortical interpositional iliac crest bone graft and talonaviculocuneiform arthrodesis completed.

- **In-situ Talonavicular Arthrodesis**: On the other hand, some surgeons perform in-situ talonavicular arthrodesis with no attempt at reduction of medial talonavicular subluxation (Lu et al. 2014).
- **Modified Talonaviculocuneiform Arthrodesis with Exacerbation of Medial Talonavicular Subluxation**: At the other extreme, some centers in China excise the lateral two-thirds of the navicular and deliberately 'squeeze' the medial navicular remnant further medially to make room for a tricortical iliac crest bone graft, which is interposed between the talar head and the middle/lateral cuneiform bone duo (Yu et al. 2012; Lu et al. 2022). Fixation extends from the talar head over the bone graft into the middle cuneiform (Lu et al. 2022) or across an unprepared TMT2 (Yu et al. 2012). An additional transverse lag screw crosses from the medial navicular remnant into either the talar head (Lu et al. 2022) or the bone graft (Yu et al. 2012). *NC1 is left untouched*. This procedure exacerbates the medial prominence of the navicular tuberosity.
- **'Hybrid 4-Joint' Arthrodesis:** In addition to triple arthrodesis, some authors additionally secure an iliac crest bone graft between a prepared talar head and lateral cuneiform, *leaving the medial and middle naviculocuneiform joints untouched*. They named their operation a '4-joint' arthrodesis (Zhang et al. 2017).
- **Selective Arthrodesis:** Use of SPECT-CT and clinical examination to help decide upon which joints to arthrodese, including the subtalar and calcaneocuboid joints (Sun et al. 2022).
- **Selective Arthrodesis According to Wong Groups**: See next Sect. 13.8 (Fig. 13.1).
- **Calcaneal Osteotomy:** Based on the concept of obligatory heel varus in Müller-Weiss disease, Li, Myerson, Monteagudo and Maceira advocate joint-preserving surgery in the form of a 'super' lateral displacement calcaneal osteotomy (Li et al. 2017).
- **Lateral Column Lengthening**: Ahmed et al. instead performed lateral column lengthening in 11 adolescent feet (Ahmed et al. 2019b).

**Conundrum**: All the above studies report good results regardless of (a) joints affected (b) severity of medial talonavicular subluxation (c) of whether it is reduced or not and (d) of extent of arthrodesis and fixation. Amongst such a plethora of different surgical recommendations, which procedure should a surgeon choose? The problem and hence the answer may well lie with establishment of an appropriate classification of the disease.

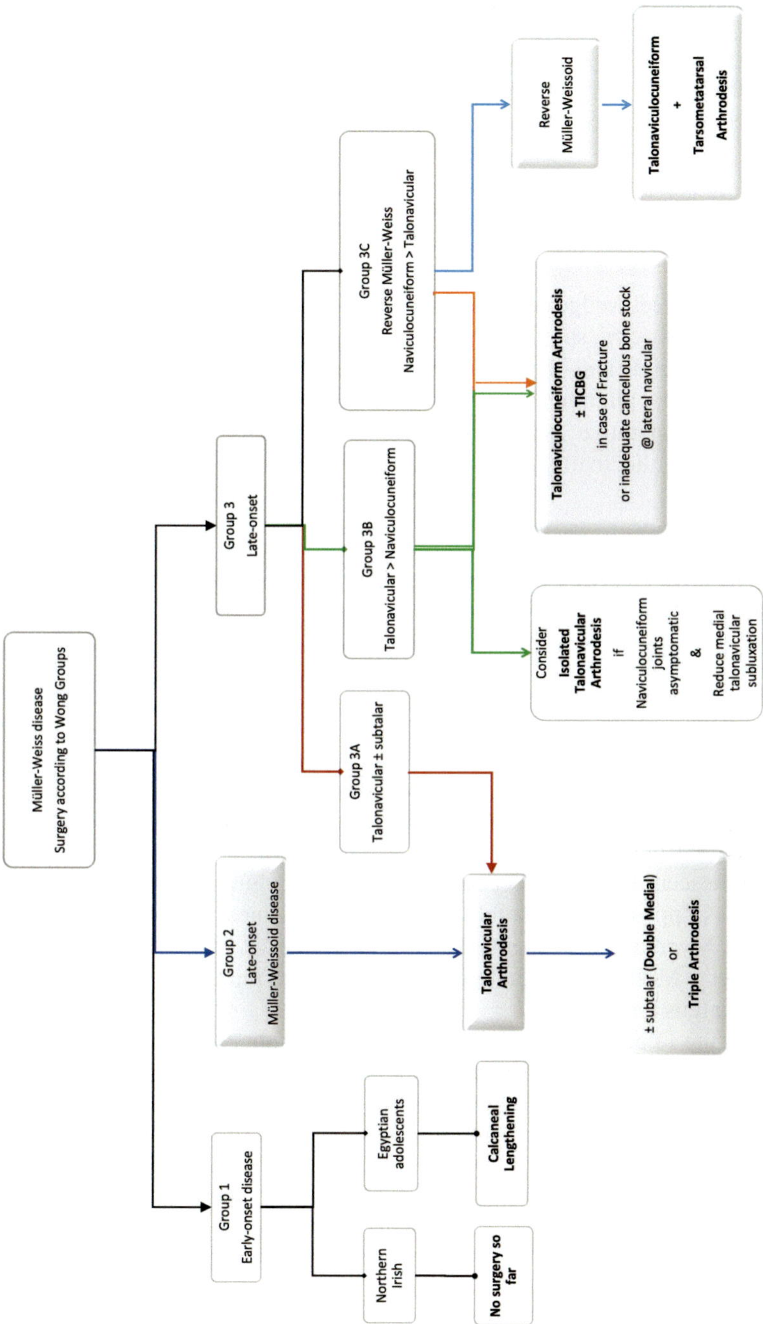


**Fig. 13.1** Surgery of Müller-Weiss disease according to Wong Groups. TICBG, tricortical iliac crest bone graft

## 13.9 Areas for Future Research in Treatment of Müller-Weiss Disease

Future research should therefore address individual groups or subgroups rather than any mixture of categories randomly lumped together.

### *13.9.1 Nonoperative Treatment of Müller-Weiss Disease*

In theory, a lateral heel wedge combined with a medial arch support as advocated by Monteagudo and Maceira, should only work when there is true heel varus (Hetsroni et al. 2007; Monteagudo and Maceira 2019). The latter may be verified radiologically by obtaining hindfoot alignment views.

Results of nonoperative treatment should be reported according to group or subgroup, and not collectively in any combination of categories.

### *13.9.2 Natural History of Group 1 Early-Onset Müller-Weiss Disease*

Maceira and Rochera had postulated that Müller-Weiss disease must originate in childhood when a cartilaginous navicular that is slow to ossify deforms under abnormal compressive stresses from an overlong second metatarsal. The young cartilage has no innervation and the child remains asymptomatic. However, any deformity persists throughout the rest of the patient's life and may become symptomatic in later life (Maceira and Rochera 2004).

The 13 adolescent Egyptian feet underwent lateral column lengthening (Ahmed et al. 2019b) as opposed to a lateral displacement calcaneal osteotomy as recommended by Li, Myerson, Monteagudo and Maceira (Li et al. 2017). They exhibited a Group 3C reverse Müller-Weiss pattern with pronounced midfoot abduction, medial arch sag and valgus heels.

In contrast, the 11 early-onset Northern Irish feet did not have the same pattern of marked midfoot abduction (Wong-Chung et al. 2023). None have required surgery at the time of publication in early 2023. That said, more recently one male patient now aged 29 years old has just presented with recent onset of painful arthritis at both talonavicular and naviculocuneiform joints and will now require talonaviculocuneiform arthrodesis. He first presented at the age of 13 years old following an injury to his left foot while using a skipping rope. His pain rapidly settled down within 6 weeks and he has not complained since until now 16 years later. It is hence conceivable that the disease does start in childhood in some cases and does not become manifest until mid to late adulthood.

Defining the natural history of early-onset Group 1 disease may actually shed more light on pathogenesis of the disease.

Geographical difference in pattern of early-onset disease may also require further research.

### 13.9.3 Group 2 Müller-Weissoid Feet

Müller-Weissoid feet are those that develop disease, mostly at the talonavicular joint, in late adulthood having had a previously normal navicular in early adulthood. Minimal to mild changes may be present at the lateral naviculocuneiform (NC3) joint but are usually asymptomatic. Fracture rarely occurs in Group 2. Surgery has consisted of talonavicular ± subtalar arthrodesis with reportedly good results (Wong-Chung et al. 2023, 2024).

Future research should confirm the satisfactory results of talonavicular ± subtalar arthrodesis, including union rates and complications. In addition, investigators will need to verify whether Maceira stage makes any difference to outcomes within that group and more importantly, if outcome is instead related to degree of correction of the medial longitudinal arch and midfoot abduction rather than to Maceira stage.

### 13.9.4 Group 3A Late-Onset Disease

Disease is limited to the talonavicular only ± subtalar joint. Fracture is rarely encountered in Group 3A. Surgery has consisted of talonavicular ± subtalar arthrodesis with reportedly good results (Wong-Chung et al. 2023, 2024).

Similarly, future studies should confirm satisfactory outcomes of talonavicular ± subtalar arthrodesis in Group 3A disease. In addition, researchers will need to clarify whether Maceira stages make any difference to outcomes within that group or if outcome is instead related to degree of correction of the medial arch and midfoot abduction rather than to Maceira stage.

### 13.9.5 Groups 3B and 3C Maceira Stages II, III and IV Without Fracture

Groups 3B and 3C affect both sides of the navicular. In Group 3B, the talonavicular is more affected than the naviculocuneiform joint, whereas the naviculocuneiform joints are more involved than the talonavicular in Group 3C disease.

In the absence of fracture and with good bone stock at the lateral navicular, treatment has consisted of talonaviculocuneiform arthrodesis with reportedly good results (Wong-Chung et al. 2023, 2024). Future studies should confirm results of talonaviculocuneiform arthrodesis in Groups 3B and 3C without associated fracture at different Maceira stages. Here again, Maceira Stages II, III or IV may not be as important in determining outcomes of surgery as degree of restoration of the medial longitudinal arch and correction of midfoot abduction, especially in the Group 3C reverse Müller-Weiss feet.

Note that in Group 3B disease, it may be possible to perform Save as many Joints as Possible (SamJap) surgery because sometimes asymptomatic degeneration affects the lateral naviculocuneiform (NC3) joint with relative sparing of the medial (NC1) and middle naviculocuneiform (NC2) joints, as also observed by Harnroongroj and Chuckpaiwong (Harnroongroj and Chuckpaiwong 2018).

However, in Group 3C, which affects the naviculocuneiform more than the talonavicular joint, it becomes necessary to perform a talonaviculocuneiform arthrodesis, fusing the naviculocuneiform articulation as well as the talonavicular joint, which is always involved ± medially subluxed.

### 13.9.6 Groups 3B and 3C Disease with Fracture

Fracture at the lateral navicular occurs in 65% of Wong Group 3B and 32% of Wong Group 3C. It may be undisplaced. In either Group 3B or Group 3C, it may progress to Maceira Stage V, which is marked by formation of the talocuneiform joint. It is formed by the talar head articulating directly with the lateral cuneiform bone, subsequent to dorsal extrusion of the lateral navicular fragment and medial subluxation at the talonavicular joint.

### 13.9.7 Group 3B Maceira Stage V Disease

A common presentation in the literature is one affecting mostly the talonavicular joint with fracture of the lateral navicular, dorsal extrusion of the lateral navicular fragment and direct articulation of the talar head with the lateral cuneiform—the 'talocuneiform' joint. The dorsally extruded navicular fragment is considered avascular and is usually excised. So, which surgery works best for this Group 3B Maceira Stage V?

(a) A more conventional joint-sacrificing approach such as talonaviculocuneiform arthrodesis with interpositional autogenous tricortical iliac crest bone graft or interpositional femoral head allograft? (Mayich 2016)

(b) Or reduce medial talonavicular subluxation using a pin distractor to derotate the navicular lateralward from its medially subluxed position and perform talonavicular arthrodesis only, preserving the naviculocuneiform joints, in a Save-as-many-Joints-as-Possible (SamJap) approach as described and advocated by Yuan et al. (Yuan et al. 2019).
(c) Or reduce medial talonavicular subluxation and still perform a talonaviculocuneiform arthrodesis as described by Bai et al. (Bai et al. 2023). After appropriate medial soft tissue release and excision of blocking osteophytes at the lateral aspect of the navicular, including at the '4-corners' as named by Doyle et al. (Doyle et al. 2012), the navicular is derotated from its displaced plantar medial location dorsalward and lateralward to its correct location at the apex of the medial longitudinal arch. This maneuver simultaneously corrects medial column length and medial arch sag. The lateral defect can then be measured and filled with an interference-fit tricortical iliac crest bone graft.
(d) Or perform a hybrid 4-joint arthrodesis as advocated by Zhang et al. (Zhang et al. 2017). It consists of a triple arthrodesis and interposition of a tricortical iliac crest bone graft between the talar head and the lateral cuneiform. NC1 and NC2 are left untouched.

### *13.9.8 Groups 3B and 3C with Undisplaced Fractures—Treat as for Stage V?*

The previous section dealt with fracture at Maceira Stage V disease in which the lateral navicular fragment is completely displaced dorsally. But once fracture occurs, whether the smaller lateral navicular fragment extrudes dorsally or remains undisplaced and aligned with the medial remnant, how much vascularity does it really have and what are its potential for union?

For Groups 3B and 3C with undisplaced fracture and no dorsal extrusion, the surgical options then are:

- Excise the lateral fragment because it is likely avascular and therefore unlikely to unite, and perform talonaviculocuneiform arthrodesis with tricortical interpositional iliac crest bone graft as per Maceira Stage V
- Or adopt a SamJap approach by reducing medial talonavicular subluxation and performing talonavicular arthrodesis only, anticipating that the fracture will heal.

The case series of Wong-Chung et al. included one patient, in whom the lateral fragment was mildly displaced in the medio-lateral plane but not in the sagittal plane (Wong-Chung et al. 2024). The authors performed a double medial arthrodesis with a retrograde compression screw across the subtalar joint and a 2-hole Uni-CP plate (Integra LifeSciences, Plainsboro, NJ) across the medial part of the talonavicular joint. Laterally, a 4-hole Uni-CP plate aimed to stabilize both the lateral part of the talonavicular joint and the 2 navicular fragments. Two screws through the distal limb of the 4-hole Uni-CP engaged one each into the medial and lateral navicular fragments, which had been apposed together after preparation of their adjoining edges. Yuan et al. had remarked that compression across the talonavicular joint may help bring in blood supply from the talar head to the navicular (Yuan et al. 2019). Likewise, Wong-Chung et al. had hoped the fragments would unite to each other and to the talar head, which had good vascularity. Union happened at neither the talonavicular joint nor between the 2 navicular fragments. Another patient developed nonunion at the talonavicular joint due to poor bone stock at the lateral navicular.

The authors concluded that talonavicular arthrodesis is not advisable in case of inadequate bone stock or fracture, even if undisplaced, through the lateral navicular.

Yamaguchi et al. performed open reduction and internal fixation of what they presumed were bipartite naviculars in two 14-year-old boys (Yamaguchi et al. 2016). As discussed in Sect. 1.8, both cases actually represented early-onset Müller-Weiss disease with fragmentation at the lateral navicular. CT scan had shown the navicular fragments to be close to each other in both patients. Despite meticulous preparation of the bone ends, bone grafting with autologous cancellous bone and seemingly encouraging signs of bone union on CT scan at 3–6 months postoperatively, both went on to painful nonunion upon resuming sports activities.

Fishman et al. performed vascularized pedicle bone grafting from either the cuboid, middle or lateral cuneiform, for 8 feet with navicular nonunions, 5 of which had osteonecrosis (Fishman et al. 2012). Of the 5, three patients were aged 20, 35 and 53 years old. The other two, aged 64 and 68 years old, had concomitant talonavicular arthritis. No further details, pre or postoperative radiographs were shown, although the authors mentioned Müller-Weiss disease twice in their introduction. Perhaps, at least the 2 feet with talonavicular degeneration had Müller-Weiss disease. All went on to unite, except for the 20-year-old, who then required revision internal fixation with iliac crest bone graft. In this study, a vascularized free pedicle graft was added to promote union between the navicular fragments.

In conclusion, once fracture of the lateral navicular occurs, even if undisplaced, this author opines it best to treat as for a Maceira Stage V lesion, excise the lateral navicular fragment and perform talonaviculocuneiform arthrodesis with interpositional tricortical iliac crest bone graft.

### *13.9.9 Lateral Displacement Calcaneal Osteotomy Alone*

Results of lateral displacement calcaneal osteotomy alone should likewise be reported according to group or subgroup, and not collectively in any combination of categories.

## 13.10 Other Surgical Unknowns to Be Answered by Future Studies

- When performing either talonavicular or talonaviculocuneiform arthrodesis, does nonreduction, reduction or degree of reduction of medial talonavicular subluxation affect outcomes? Sects. 7.6, 7.7 and 7.8 dealt with techniques of achieving reduction by medial soft tissue release and clearance of lateral blockages. Future studies should measure and state degree of correction of medial talonavicular subluxation.
- When should arthrodesis be extended to the naviculocuneiform joints? By definition, always in Group 3C and never for Group 3A. In Group 2 and Group 3B, mild asymptomatic degeneration may be encountered at NC3 and can be safely left alone, as it has not been seen to progress to such extent as to require further surgical intervention (Harnroongroj and Chuckpaiwong 2018; Wong-Chung et al. 2024). In Group 3B, extension to talonaviculocuneiform arthrodesis is indicated in case of symptomatic degeneration at the naviculocuneiform joints as assessed by SPECT-CT ± diagnostic injection and in case of fracture at the lateral navicular as already discussed in Sect. 13.9.8.
- And should all or which of the 3 naviculocuneiform (NC) joints be included in a talonaviculocuneiform arthrodesis?
  - Beginning with Fernández de Retana et al. (2004), some surgeons such as Yuan et al. (2019) and Cao et al. (2012, 2017) have followed suit and included only NC1 leaving NC2 and NC3 untouched.
  - Other surgeons like Yu et al. (2012), Lu et al. (2022) and Liu et al. (2022) include NC2 and NC3 and leave NC1 untouched. To make room for tricortical iliac crest bone grafts between the talar head and the middle/lateral cuneiform bone duo, the first two centers maximally displace the medial navicular remnant, raising concern about undue medial prominence.
  - On the other hand, Zhang et al. prepare NC3 only and leave NC1 and NC2 untouched (Zhang et al. 2017). Subluxation usually occurs at the talonavicular and not at the naviculocuneiform joint. As long as there is no marked residual talonavicular subluxation, application of this technique in Group 3B Stage V disease may deserve further investigation. It may also prove useful in Group 3B at stages other than Stage V in which mostly the lateral naviculocuneiform rather than NC1 and NC2 joints are involved. It preserves NC1 and NC2, which Wong-Chung et al., Harnroongroj and Chuckpaiwong have also noted to be largely intact in Müller-Weiss disease (Harnroongroj and Chuckpaiwong 2018; Wong-Chung et al. 2024).

## 13.11 Other Tools for Future Research in Müller-Weiss Disease

Other ancillary tools can help advance understanding of pathogenesis, pathomechanism and pattern of deformity in Müller-Weiss disease.

### *13.11.1 Weight-Bearing CT (WBCT)*

Although wider availability of WBCT is still wanting, it may eventually provide greater insight into why lateral shift of the talar head does not always translate into heel varus in as much as 66% of cases (Wong-Chung et al. 2021).

It will first serve to ascertain whether heel varus is an obligatory finding across all groups of Müller-Weiss disease. It may well be that the heel is in varus in certain groups or subgroups, yet in neutral or valgus in others. The WBCT windows can be adjusted to provide different kinds of images. Thus, images obtained via a Skin window will correspond to heel position as assessed clinically, whereas images acquired via X-Ray Sharp or Bone windows will give true position of the heel bone (See Sect. 3.6). Correlation between assessment by Skin versus X-Ray Sharp or Bone images would explain the discrepancy often encountered amongst clinicians in assessment and reporting heel positions not just in Müller-Weiss disease, but also in all other conditions.

Furthermore, in the same way as WBCT has shown abnormal motion at the various facets of the subtalar joint in progressive collapsing foot deformity, it may reveal what really occurs at the anterior, middle and posterior facets of the subtalar joint as the talar head moves laterally. Perhaps again, by adjusting the soft tissue windows, it may provide information on the role of the various perinavicular ligaments in the deformation process.

### *13.11.2 Pedobarography*

Similarly, pedobarographic analysis by group may prove more informative than collectively in any combination of groups and subgroups.

Hetsroni et al. performed pedography in 8 feet, all of which were said to have advanced radiographic changes (Hetsroni et al. 2007). They found raised pressures at the midfoot and decreased plantar pressures at the forefoot and medial heel. As a result, nonoperative treatment of Müller-Weiss disease consists of a lateral heel wedge and a medial arch support, regardless of group and actual heel position. And some surgeons advocate lateral displacement calcaneal osteotomy alone regardless of disease group and preserve all the foot joints. These findings hence need verification according to group and subgroup.

## 13.12 Navicular Replacement

Angthong et al. (Thailand, 2023) proposed a new treatment algorithm based on Maceira stages (Angthong et al. 2023). For Maceira Stages I-II, calcaneal osteotomy or lengthening may be considered in cases of mild to moderate compression of the lateral navicular. For more severe compression, the authors ask to consider either arthrodesis of the arthritic joints or a navicular prosthesis in the second limb of their decision flowchart. For Maceira Stage III-IV not involving the ankle, the third limb recommends triple, talonavicular or talonaviculocuneiform arthrodesis ± subtalar arthrodesis. The fourth limb pertains to disease involving the ankle joint, when either tibiotalocalcaneal arthrodesis or total ankle replacement may be considered.

Firstly, by definition, there is no radiological evidence of compression in Stage I. Neither calcaneal osteotomy nor lengthening nor arthrodesis nor prosthesis is appropriate for Maceira Stage I disease.

Secondly, the authors' criteria for a navicular replacement are an intact articular cartilage at both the talonavicular and naviculocuneiform articulations. However, while the naviculocuneiform joint may escape degeneration in some cases, arthritis nearly always occurs at the talonavicular joint, which equates to arthritic damage of the talar head.

Thirdly, while navicular replacement has been reported for osteonecrosis following trauma, there is no report of its application in Müller-Weiss disease. The latter condition is a chronic and not an acute disease like trauma. In Müller-Weiss disease, scarring as noted by Nelson and Rivello and loss of column lengths result from compression and fragmentation of the lateral navicular (Nelson and Rivello 2012). Using the contralateral normal navicular as template for manufacturing a navicular prosthesis will not take into account the degree of soft tissue contracture and bone loss (Angthong et al. 2019; Adams and Danilkowicz 2021). Difficulty may then arise inserting the component in a very tight contracted space.

Fourthly, it does not address the biomechanical factors that caused osteonecrosis of the navicular in the first place, namely overlength of the second metatarsal. Perhaps, any future endeavours to utilize a navicular replacement should consider shortening metatarsal osteotomies as an adjunct.

### Concluding Remarks—Epilogue

Although recognition of Müller-Weiss disease is increasing through greater awareness, sample size of most studies published so far remains small due to relative rarity of the condition. It will decrease even further once investigators are required to publish their results according to group or subgroup. Nevertheless, it is essential to compare likes with likes. In order to evaluate efficacy of various surgical interventions for a particular category of feet, multi-center studies may be the way to obtaining sufficient numbers for statistical significance.

To define gold standards in treatment, a common platform first needs to be established. With time and testing, other scholars will refine and fine-tune the suggested combined classifications through additions, subtractions or alterations. Until then and towards that goal, future studies should state (1) the Wong Group (2) the Maceira stage according to lateral Méary's angle (3) treatment applied and degree of correction of medial talonavicular subluxation. Parameters included in the combined grouping system of Wong-Chung et al. and staging system of Maceira are (a) age at onset (b) documentation of a previous radiologically normal navicular (c) joints affected (d) the dorsoplantar talo-first metatarsal angle (5) lateral Méary's angle (6) presence of fracture and (7) heel varus as measured on hindfoot alignment view.

This book, especially this last chapter, will hopefully have stimulated interest and opened up numerous avenues for research into the unknowns of Müller-Weiss disease. This may perforce necessitate and encourage national and international collaboration. Only through a standardized platform will physicians then be able to advise and recommend the best treatment in an evidence-based fashion. It will all be for the benefit of the young and older sufferers with this condition.

## References

Adams SB, Danilkowicz RM. Talonavicular joint-sparing 3D printed navicular replacement for osteonecrosis of the navicular. Foot Ankle Int. 2021;42(9):1197–204. https://doi.org/10.1177/10711007211002807.

Ahmed ASAA, Kandil MI, Tabl EA, Elgazzar AS. Müller-Weiss disease: a topical review. Foot Ankle Int. 2019a;40(12):1447–57. https://doi.org/10.1177/1071100719877000.

Ahmed AA, Kandil MI, Tabl EA. Preliminary outcomes of calcaneal lengthening in adolescent flatfoot in Müller-Weiss disease. Foot Ankle Int. 2019b;40(7):803–7. https://doi.org/10.1177/1071100719833928

Angthong C, Stufkens SAS, Rajbhandari P. The navicular prosthesis template: a cadaveric study of the talonavicular morphometric profiles and side-to-side differences. Foot Ankle Orthop. 2019;4(4). https://doi.org/10.1177/2473011419S00096

Angthong C, Younger ASE, Chuckpaiwong B, Harnroongroj T, Veljkovic A. A novel update on the management of Müller-Weiss disease: presentation of a treatment algorithm. Cartilage. 2023:19476035231205684. https://doi.org/10.1177/19476035231205684. Epub ahead of print.

Bai W, Li Y, Shen G, Zhang H, Li X, Zhu Y. Talonavicular-cuneiform arthrodesis for the treatment of Müller-Weiss: mid-term results of 15 cases after 5 years. BMC Musculoskelet Disord. 2023;24:178. https://doi.org/10.1186/s12891-023-06293-1.

Bateman JK. Broken hock in the greyhound. Repair methods and the plastic scaphoid. Vet Res. 1958;70:621–3.

Brailsford JF. Osteochondritis of the adult tarsal navicular. J Bone Joint Surg. 1939;21(1):111–20.

Cao HH, Tang K-L, Xu J-Z. Peri-navicular arthrodesis for the stage III Müller-Weiss disease. Foot Ankle Int. 2012;33(6):475–8. https://doi.org/10.3113/FAI.2012.0475.

Cao HH, Lu WZ, Tang KL. Isolated talonavicular arthrodesis and talonavicular-cuneiform arthrodesis for the Müller-Weiss disease. J Orthop Surg Res. 2017;12(83):1–6. https://doi.org/10.1186/s13018-017-0581-4.

Chang SM, Chen PY, Tsai MS, Shee BW. Light bulb procedure for the treatment of tarsal navicular osteonecrosis after failed percutaneous decompression: a case report. J Foot Ankle Surg. 2019;58(1):187–91. https://doi.org/10.1053/j.jfas.2018.08.003.

Chiavegatti R, Canales P, Saldias E, Isidro A. Earliest probable case of Mueller-Weiss disease from ancient Egypt. J Foot Ankle Surg. 2018;57(5):1034–6. https://doi.org/10.1053/j.jfas.2018.03.004.

Coris EE, Lombardo JA. Tarsal navicular stress fractures. Am Fam Physician. 2003;67(1):85–90.

Cullen NP, Singh D, Clowry O, Dudkiewicz I. Symptomatic non-union of second metatarsal stress fracture following talo-navicular arthrodesis. Foot Ankle Surg. 2005;11(4):203–5. https://doi.org/10.1016/j.fas.2005.07.001.

Doyle T, Napier RJ, Wong-Chung J. Recognition and management of Müller-Weiss disease. Foot Ankle Int. 2012;33(4):275–81. https://doi.org/10.3113/FAI.2012.0275.

Fernández de Retana P, Maceira E, Fernández-Valencia JA, Suso S. Arthrodesis of the talonavicular-cuneiform joints in Müller-Weiss disease. Foot Ankle Clin. 2004;9(1):65–72. https://doi.org/10.1016/S1083-7515(03)00175-X

Fishman FG, Adams SB, Easley ME, Nunley JA. Vascularized pedicle bone grafting for nonunions of the tarsal navicular. Foot Ankle Int. 2012;33:734–9. https://doi.org/10.3113/FAI.2012.0734.

Fitch KD, Blackwell JB, Gilmour WN. Operation for non-union of stress fracture of the tarsal navicular. J Bone Joint Surg [br]. 1989;71(1):105–10. https://doi.org/10.1302/0301-620X.71B1.2644288.

Fornaciari P, Gilgen A, Zwicky L, Horn Lang T, Hintermann B. Isolated talonavicular fusion with tension band for Müller-Weiss syndrome. Foot Ankle Int. 2014;35(12):1316–22. https://doi.org/10.1177/1071100714548197.

Goergen TG, Venn-Watson EA, Rossman DJ, Resnick D, Gerber KH. Tarsal navicular stress fractures in runners. AJR Am J Roentgenol. 1981;136(1):201–3. https://doi.org/10.2214/ajr.136.1.201.

Harnroongroj T, Chuckpaiwong B. Müller-Weiss disease: three- to eight-year follow-up outcomes of isolated talonavicular arthrodesis. J Foot Ankle Surg. 2018;57(5):1014–9. https://doi.org/10.1053/j.jfas.2018.01.008.

Harnroongroj T, Tharmviboonsri T, Chuckpaiwong B. Müller-Weiss disease: the descriptive factors of failure conservative treatment. Foot Ankle Int. 2021;42(8):1022–30. https://doi.org/10.1177/10711007211002826

Hermena S, Francis M. Clinical presentation, imaging features, and management of Müller-Weiss disease. Cureus. 2021;13(10): e18659. https://doi.org/10.7759/cureus.18659.

Hetsroni I, Nyska M, Ayalon M. Plantar pressure distribution in patients with Müller-Weiss disease. Foot Ankle Int. 2007;28(2):237–41. https://doi.org/10.3113/FAI.2007.0237.

Hunter LY. Stress fracture of the tarsal navicular. More frequent than we realize? Am J Sports Med. 1981;9(4):217–9. https://doi.org/10.1177/036354658100900405

Li S-Y, Myerson MS, Monteagudo M, Maceira E. Efficacy of calcaneus osteotomy for treatment of symptomatic Müller-Weiss disease. Foot Ankle Int. 2017;38(3):261–9. https://doi.org/10.1177/1071100716677741.

Liu W, Chen Y, Zeng G, Yang T, Ma M, Song W. Individual surgical treatment of stage IV Müller-Weiss disease according to CT/MRI examination: a retrospective study of 12 cases. Front Surg. 2022;17(9): 694597. https://doi.org/10.3389/fsurg.2022.694597.

Lu CK, Fu YC, Cheng YM, Huang PJ. Isolated talonavicular arthrodesis for Müller-Weiss disease. Kaohsiung J Med Sci. 2014;30(9):471–6. https://doi.org/10.1016/j.kjms.2014.05.001.

Lu L, Liu B, Zeng J, Chen W, Hu F, Ma Q, Yu G. Efficacy of triple and talonavicular arthrodesis for the treatment of III-V Müller-Weiss disease. Tohoku J Exp Med. 2022;258(2):97–102. https://doi.org/10.1620/tjem.2022.J062.

Maceira E, Rochera R. Müller-Weiss disease: clinical and biomechanical features. Foot Ankle Clin. 2004;9(1):105–25. https://doi.org/10.1016/S1083-7515(03)00153-0.

Mann JA, Pedowitz DI. Evaluation and treatment of navicular stress fractures, including nonunions, revision surgery, and persistent pain after treatment. Foot Ankle Clin. 2009;14(2):187–204. https://doi.org/10.1016/j.fcl.2009.01.003.

Manoli AII, Graham B. The subtle cavus foot, "the underpronator", a review. Foot Ankle Int. 2005;26(3):256–63.

Manoli AII, Smith DG, Hansen ST Jr. Scarred muscle excision for the treatment of established ischemic contracture of the lower extremity. Clin Orthop. 1993;292:309–14.

Mayich DJ. The treatment of Mueller-Weiss disease: a systematic approach. Tech Foot Ankle Surg. 2016;15(2):59–73. https://doi.org/10.1097/BTF.0000000000000088.

McKeon KE, McCormick JJ, Johnson JE, Klein SE. Intraosseous and extraosseous arterial anatomy of the adult navicular. Foot Ankle Int. 2012;33(10):857–61. https://doi.org/10.3113/FAI.2012.0857.

Mohiuddin T, Jennison T, Damany D. Müller-Weiss disease—review of current knowledge. Foot Ankle Surg. 2014;20(2):79–84. https://doi.org/10.1016/j.fas.2013.11.001.

Molina WF, Nogueira MP, Alvo FS, Heitzmann LG. Müller-Weiss disease: a functional and quality of life assessment. Int Orthop. 2023;47(8):1921–7. https://doi.org/10.1007/s00264-023-05851-5.

Monteagudo M, Maceira E. Management of Müller-Weiss disease. Foot Ankle Clin. 2019;24(1):89–105. https://doi.org/10.1016/j.fcl.2018.09.006.

Monteagudo M, Martínez-de-Albornoz P. Navicular fracture. Foot Ankle Clin. 2022;27(2):457–74. https://doi.org/10.1016/j.fcl.2021.11.024

Müller W. Über eine eigenartige doppelseitige veränderung des os naviculare beim Erwachsenen [On an odd double-sided change of the tarsal navicular]. Deutsche Zeitschrift Für Chirurgie Leipzig. 1927;201:84–7.

Myerson MS. Correction of flatfoot deformity in the adult. In Reconstructive foot and ankle surgery: management of complications, vol. 18, 2nd ed. Philadelphia:Elsevier Saunders. p. 201.

Nelson EW, Rivello GJ. Müller-Weiss disease of the tarsal navicular: an idiopathic case. J Foot Ankle Surg. 2012;51(5):636–41. https://doi.org/10.1053/j.jfas.2012.04.002.

Pavlov H, Torg JS, Freiberger RH. Tarsal navicular stress fractures: radiographic evaluation. Radiology. 1983;148(3):641–5. https://doi.org/10.1148/radiology.148.3.6224230.

Saltzman CL, el-Khoury GY. The hindfoot alignment view. Foot Ankle Int. 1995;16(9):572–6. https://doi.org/10.1177/107110079501600911

Saxena A, Fullem B, Hannaford D. Results of treatment of 22 navicular stress fractures and a new proposed radiographic classification system. J Foot Ankle Surg. 2000;39(2):96–103. https://doi.org/10.1016/s1067-2516(00)80033-2.

Sun C, Ebben B, Li S, Zhu M, Myerson MS, Zhang M-Z. The use of SPECT-CT to define treatment for Müller-Weiss disease: a prospective radiographic and clinical study. Foot Ankle Orthop. 2022;7(4). https://doi.org/10.1177/2473011421S00958

Tan A, Smulders YC, Zöphel OT. Use of remodeled femoral head allograft for tarsal reconstruction in the treatment of Müller-Weiss disease. J Foot Ankle Surg. 2011;50(6):721–6. https://doi.org/10.1053/j.jfas.2011.04.043.

Tanaka Y, Takakura Y, Omokawa S, Kumai T, Sugimoto K. Crank-shaped arthrodesis for a flatfoot with a bipartite navicular: a case report. Foot Ankle Int. 2006;27(9):734–7. https://doi.org/10.1177/107110070602700914.

Tile M. Pelvic fractures—should they be fixed. J Bone Joint Surg. 1988;70B:1–12. https://doi.org/10.1302/0301-620X.70B1.3276697.

Tile M. Fractures of the pelvis and acetabulum. 2nd ed. Baltimore, MD: Williams & Wilkins; 1995. p. 3.

Toren AJ, Hahn DB, Brown WC, Stone PA, Ng A. Vascularized scapular free bone graft after nonunion of a tarsal navicular stress fracture: a case report. J Foot Ankle Surg. 2013;52(2):221–6. https://doi.org/10.1053/j.jfas.2012.12.010.

Torg JS, Pavlov H, Cooley LH, Bryant MH, Arnoczky SP, Bergfeld J, Hunter LY. Stress fractures of the tarsal navicular. A retrospective review of twenty-one cases. J Bone Joint Surg [Am]. 1982;64(5):700–12.

Tosun B, Al F, Tosun A. Spontaneous osteonecrosis of the tarsal navicular in an adult: Mueller-Weiss syndrome. J Foot Ankle Surg. 2011;50(2):221–4. https://doi.org/10.1053/j.jfas.2010.10.019.

Towne LC, Blazina ME, Cozen LN. Fatigue fracture of the tarsal navicular. J Bone Joint Surg [am]. 1970;52(2):376–8.

Volk C. Zwei fälle von os naviculare pedis bipartitum. Z Orthop Ihre Grenzgeb. 1937;66:396–403.

Weiss K. Über die "malazie" des os naviculare pedis [On the malacia of the tarsal navicular]. Fortschr Geb Rontgenstr. 1927;45:63–7.

Wong-Chung J, McKenna R, Tucker A, Gibson D, Datta P. Radiographic analysis of Müller-Weiss disease. Foot Ankle Surg. 2021;27(5):501–9. https://doi.org/10.1016/j.fas.2020.06.009.

Wong-Chung J, Walls A, Lynch-Wong M, Cassidy R, McKenna R, Wilson A, Stephens M. Towards understanding Müller-Weiss disease from an analysis of 95 cases. Foot Ankle Surg. 2023;29(5):401–11. https://doi.org/10.1016/j.fas.2023.05.004.

Wong-Chung J, Blythe A, Lynch-Wong M, McKenna R, Wilson A, Stephens M. Outcomes of Selective Arthrodesis Based on Joints Affected in 33 Feet with Müller-Weiss Disease. J Foot Ankle Surg. 2024;63(2):199–206. https://doi.org/10.1053/j.jfas.2023.11.001

Yamaguchi S, Niki H, Akagi R, Yamamoto Y, Sasho T. Failure of internal fixation for painful bipartite navicular in two adolescent soccer players: a report of two cases. J Foot Ankle Surg. 2016;55(6):1323–6. https://doi.org/10.1053/j.jfas.2016.01.015.

Yu G, Zhao Y, Zhou J, Zhang M. Fusion of talonavicular and naviculocuneiform joints for the treatment of Müller-Weiss disease. J Foot Ankle Surg. 2012;51(4):415–9. https://doi.org/10.1053/j.jfas.2012.04.004.

Yuan C, Wang C, Zhang C, Huang J, Wang X, Ma X. Derotation of the talus and arthrodesis treatment of stages II-V Müller-Weiss disease: Midterm results of 36 cases. Foot Ankle Int. 2019;40(5):506–14. https://doi.org/10.1177/1071100719829457.

Zhang H, Li J, Qiao Y, Yu J, Cheng Y, Liu Y, Gao C, Li J. Open triple fusion versus TNC arthrodesis in the treatment of Mueller-Weiss disease. J Orthop Surg Res. 2017;12:13. https://doi.org/10.1186/s13018-017-0513-3.

Zhang M-Z, Yu G. Surgical treatment for Müller-Weiss disease. Foot Ankle Orthop. 2018;3(3). https://doi.org/10.1177/2473011418S00536

# Index



© The Editor(s) (if applicable) and The Author(s), under exclusive license to Springer Nature Switzerland AG 2024

J. Wong-Chung, *Comprehensive Guide to Müller-Weiss Disease*,
https://doi.org/10.1007/978-3-031-66644-5

MIX
Papier aus verantwortungsvollen Quellen
Paper from responsible sources
FSC® C105338

If you have any concerns about our products,
you can contact us on
**ProductSafety@springernature.com**

In case Publisher is established outside the EU,
the EU authorized representative is:
**Springer Nature Customer Service Center GmbH**
**Europaplatz 3, 69115 Heidelberg, Germany**

Printed by Libri Plureos GmbH
in Hamburg, Germany